GERRY BROOKS

ULTIMATE RECOVERY FROM BRAIN INJURY

A Guide to Create Your Personal Recovery Lifestyle

Ultimate Recovery From Brain Injury:
A Guide to Create Your Personal Recovery Lifestyle
Published by Sound Mind Media
Poughkeepsie, NY

ISBN: 979-8-218-45423-4 (paperback)

HEALTH & FITNESS / Diseases & Conditions / Brain

Cover and interior design by Asya Blue, copyright owned by Gerry Brooks.

DISCLAIMER: There is nothing in this book that is intended to substitute for the advice of your doctor or other licensed medical practitioner.

QUANTITY PURCHASES: Schools, companies, professional groups, clubs, and other organizations may qualify for special terms when ordering quantities of this title. For information, email hal9600@aol.com.

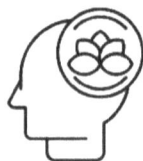

SOUND MIND
MEDIA

TABLE OF CONTENTS

DEDICATION

This book is dedicated to survivors of brain injury caused by trauma, stroke, oxygen deprivation, overdose, infection, or any other cause. It is for people who have been lawyers, housekeepers, soldiers, clerics, and short-order cooks; for people of means and those with none; for those who have been healthy their whole lives and those who have had to contend with addiction, mental illness, and other problems. This book is also dedicated to those injured indirectly—the loved ones who have been traumatized too and who also need recovery.

Finally, this book is dedicated to my colleagues in healthcare, those who also are privileged to work with patients and families recovering from brain injury—doctors, nurses, therapists, social workers, educators—and others who directly or indirectly help survivors of brain injury to find their way.

The contents of this book may also be of use to you personally. It has been my experience that we often neglect our own recovery, our own journey to best mental and physical health, which is our most important credential for doing this work and without which we are truly the blind leading the blind.

Reflection: Have your loved ones been injured too? Do they need recovery? Do you have any role to play in *their* recovery?

Disclaimer

There is nothing in this book that is intended to substitute for the advice of your doctor or other licensed medical and mental health practitioner. Where there is any discrepancy, please consult with your doctor or other licensed medical and mental health practitioner.

ACKNOWLEDGMENTS

This book was over ten years in the writing. There are so many who offered encouragement, insight, and assistance during that time that I am sure I cannot recall them all here. I truly regret that.

But here are a few of them: To my former boss and founder of the Northeast Center for Rehabilitation & Brain Injury, an inspired and inspirational leader, the late Anthony Salerno. To my lifelong friend, confidante, and editing consultant, Kathy Brown. To my former coworker and friend, Dr. Ron Goldman. To my former coworker and fellow author, Holly Huppert. To my publishing consultant at My Word Publishing, Amanda Miller. To my editor, Angela Renkoski. To Asya Blue Design. To Kevin Scutt, Oliver Vaughn, and Jared Whiteford. To my spiritual teachers, Koshin Paley Ellison and Robert Chodo Campbell. And to my former adviser and mentor, the renowned Nathan Zasler, MD.

And finally, and, of course, to my loving wife, Deb, who has encouraged me, put up with me, and kept me fed and *loved*.

PREFACE

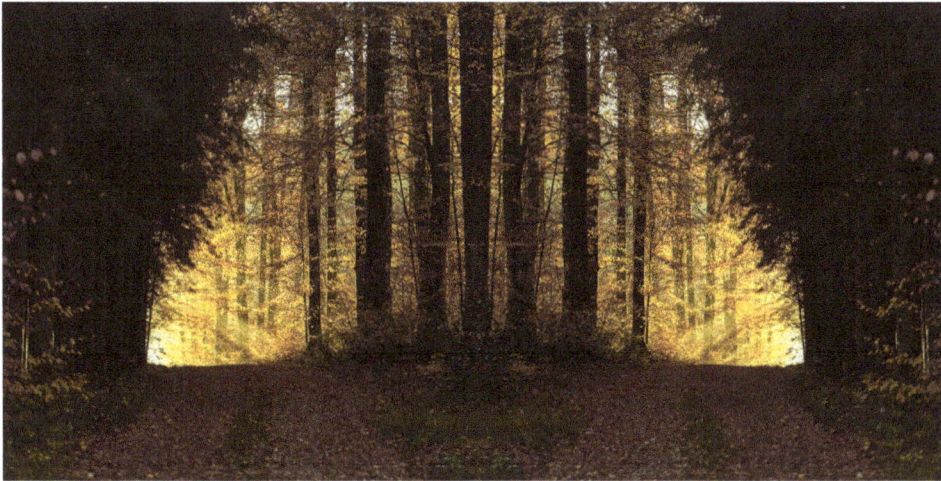

"I shall be telling this with a sigh
Somewhere ages and ages hence:
Two roads diverged in a wood, and I—
I took the one less traveled by,
And that has made all the difference."

—From "The Road Not Taken" by Robert Frost

The road (almost) not taken. Working in the field of brain injury was the only thing I was sure I *didn't* want to do by the time I completed my graduate training in speech-language pathology in 1979. I had had enough experience with it during my various internships to make this decision. It was too sad a business, and it hurt just to be around such tragedy. But fate can be fickle. Here I sit having spent most of my adult life devoted to individuals and their families dealing with the consequences of a brain injury.

I would not trade these years for anything. The pain I first encountered as a young professional so long ago, and many times since, I regard now as a sacred gift. Faced with being overcome with a grief I have had to confront almost every working day for nearly forty years, I have been forced again and again to peer deeply into myself to clarify what really makes my life worth living—and to look outward to investigate scientific and spiritual resources in order to find my own path to best mental and physical health. This book, therefore, is the culmination of this journey to date and the ideas and practices that developed along the way.

The inspiration for this book was work I did facilitating a group at the Northeast Center for Rehabilitation & Brain Injury, a 280-bed, post-acute rehabilitation center in Upstate New York. Founded in 1999 by the late Anthony Salerno, the center is dedicated to the recovery of individuals with brain injury. I served for twenty-five years, from the facility's inception, as the program director. In this capacity, and during my previous twenty years in private practice, I had the opportunity to treat scores of brain injury survivors and their families. It is fair to say that each of these individuals contributed in some way to the writing of this book. Some have been among my most profound teachers. My hope is that this work does honor to them.

INTRODUCTION

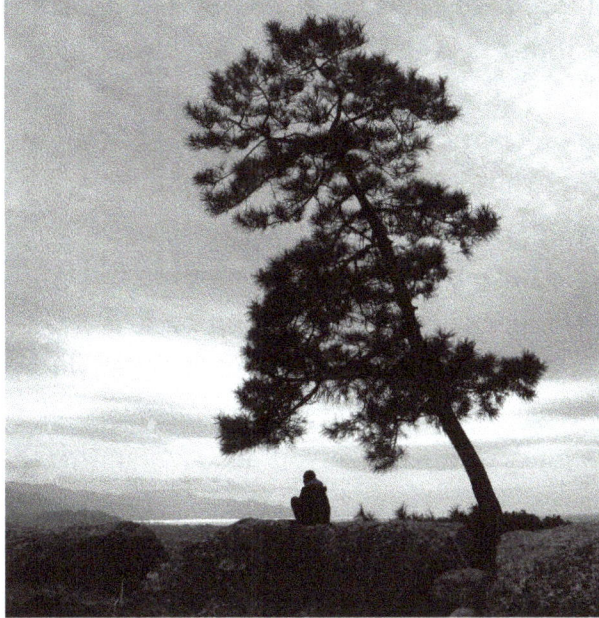

"You don't understand." In these many years working in the field of brain injury with literally thousands of survivors and their families, I have heard this statement many, many times—"You don't understand." Each time I hear it, I am humbled. It is certainly true. I *don't* understand what you have been through. I know only that you have been through a terrible ordeal that no one could have been prepared for. I also know that *any* emotions you have at this time are justified.

Disability, especially a sudden disabling condition like a brain injury, is catastrophic. Everything changes. Loss seems to be everywhere. A person's very identity shifts. No longer are they father, mother, brother, sister, breadwinner, bus driver, CEO, or basketball champ. They are, at least at first, a patient, a dependent, a receiver of care. They are trapped in a social safety net—if they're lucky. Many fall through the openings in the net and exist in a void where services, friends, family, finances, and opportunities are few or nonexistent.

I know that the anger, fear, outrage, pain, despair, hopelessness, and many other emotions you may be experiencing are natural and *necessary*. These emotions represent nothing less than your strong emotional connection with Life, emotions that result from missing things you value and want, and from desiring something better than what you feel you have right now. *These are the emotions out of which recovery is made.* In fact, without them, what I refer to as Ultimate Recovery would not be possible.

There are so many catastrophes that can and do occur in people's lives, and medical science has learned a good deal about how people survive such events. We know, for example, that human beings are tremendously resilient, and at some point, the vast majority of people heal, not just physically but emotionally and spiritually too. In some cases it happens slowly, beginning with a faint voice from within that murmurs now and then, a voice that is muffled and not easily understood at first. It might be a voice filled with anger, but it is not the voice of a victim—it is a stronger, more certain, more determined voice. *It is the voice of a survivor.*

Perhaps you are beginning to hear that voice. If so, it is important to try to understand that the emotions you feel do not indicate your life is over, but that, in fact, you may be ready to begin a new one.

You might be thinking about time you have lost to your injury; time you would have been working and earning a living; time you would have spent with your spouse, with children or grandchildren; time tending a garden, hunting, cooking, playing a sport, making art, writing, or playing music; time you would have been doing any number of things had you not been injured. Perhaps you are beginning to experience an overwhelming urgency to make up for this lost time, to get back to your life, your job, your children, your friends, your home. This too is good, for *once harnessed, this is the energy that will fuel your recovery.*

I hope you picked up this book not because you are sick and tired—but because you are sick and tired *of being sick and tired.* If so, read on. There is something here for you.

This book is not about getting back what you had before the injury. Recovery defined in terms of going back is doomed to failure and unending grief. It is never possible to go back. It is only possible to go forward. But this book is not about passive "acceptance" or about accepting the unacceptable. This book is about setting the bar high and aspiring to what most people want but few achieve: a good and healthy life.

You are not your injury. There is more, much more, to anyone than a single event in their lives. So this book is not just about recovering from a brain injury. It is about the challenge we all share to live meaningfully and develop capacities we all possess to meet that challenge. In the pages that follow, we will explore some of what it takes to be whole, happy, healthy, resilient, satisfied, and content; in other words, what it takes to achieve and sustain best mental and physical health. If your recovery doesn't add up to this, what's the point?

Ultimate Recovery is not a final destination or outcome. No one who exercises or diets expects that once they reach their goal, they can stop exercising and stop watching their diet. In that same way, meeting the challenge of living is not about reaching some final destination or outcome. The title of this book, *Ultimate Recovery,* refers to discovering what it takes to feel good and doing it—*for the rest of your life.*

First, the bad news. Ultimate Recovery is going to cost you. "You become what you practice" will be one of our mottos. Practice is the cost of Ultimate Recovery, and practice is the focus of this book. I will present seven specific practices. There are other chapters devoted to related topics that I hope are helpful as well.

The good news. Ultimate Recovery is definitely within your grasp. In fact, you can't fail—if you don't quit. That's another of our mottos. Just get started. Don't stress. Proceed at your own pace.

I'm confident there is something here of benefit for you.

How to use this book. I recommend that you take your time moving through this book. Remember that we are embarking on a change of lifestyle and such a change must happen over a lifetime. Be prepared to read and reflect, read and reflect, read and reflect. You will face many obstacles along the way and it won't be easy. But there is no rush and the long-term rewards will be substantial. Just commit to taking your time and to not quitting.

OVERVIEW OF ULTIMATE RECOVERY

WHAT IT IS

- Ultimate Recovery is not about going back but going forward to achieve and sustain a lifestyle that promotes best mental and physical health.
- Ultimate Recovery is the foundation of a healthy lifestyle that, once established, will allow you to pursue other goals and create a life worth living.
- Ultimate Recovery is a lifestyle that will allow you to recover again and again after any of the setbacks we all experience during our lifetime.

WHAT IT'S NOT

- It won't detract from any other goal or responsibility you have. On the contrary, it will vastly increase your ability to meet any other goal and fulfill any other responsibility.
- It's not selfish. The time you will be devoting to yourself is the least selfish thing you can do. If you manage to feel better and do better, who is that bad for? No one. Who is that good for? Everyone.

YOU DESERVE TO RECOVER

- You didn't deserve to be injured, no matter how it happened.
- You do deserve to recover and live a healthy, satisfying life.
- You can do it, no matter what you've done until now and no matter how long you've been doing it. If you are now willing to give yourself the attention you deserve, you will succeed.

ULTIMATE RECOVERY IS POSSIBLE

- If you adopt the practices recommended, you will become healthier, a little at a time.
- But remember: Ultimate Recovery is not a one-time achievement; it is a lifestyle.
- You will become what you practice.

IT WILL REQUIRE CHANGE

- Most people have never received training in how to live a healthy life.
- Change will be necessary to replace old habits with some new ones.
- This book focuses on seven lifestyle management practices around which to build an intentional, mentally and physically healthy lifestyle.

YOU ARE THE ULTIMATE DECIDER

- Don't be convinced or deterred by others—only you can decide.
- First learn and try the practices described in this book.
- Then decide if they can work for you.

You Can't Fail If You Don't Quit.

SECTION 1

ELIMINATING BARRIERS TO RECOVERY

CHAPTER 1

CONDUCTING A PERSONAL INVENTORY

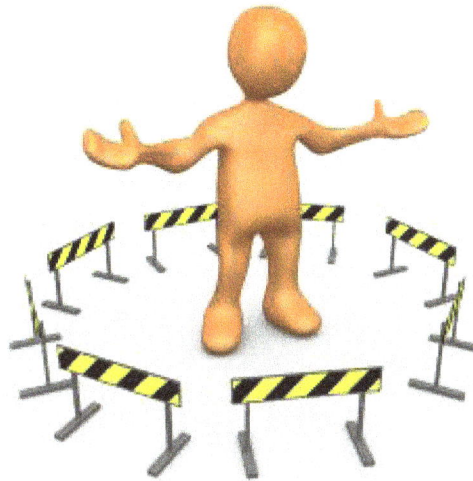

Getting started. Ultimate Recovery begins with understanding that Life is unpredictable, uncontrollable, and ever-changing. Your injury is one example of this, and there are many examples in everyone's lives if we stop to think about them. But though it's true that we can't control the circumstances of our life, we often can control how we live with those circumstances.

How you live is what we call lifestyle. If we are maintaining a generally healthy lifestyle, it will be much easier to right the boat after being capsized by one of Life's unpredictable waves. So a healthy lifestyle is a kind of remedy for Life's ills.

A healthy lifestyle that leads to your best mental and physical health—what we call Ultimate Recovery—is the result of maintaining a routine organized around three main life activities: things we *have* to do, things we *love* to do, and the *7 Recovery Practices* that are the subject of future chapters. Each of these practices is an integral part of the formula, and each one supports and strengthens the others. There is no perfecting any of them; there is only practice. I like to say, "Practice *is* perfection," because you can't fail if you never quit practicing.

Exercise: Clearing the Way. It's important to clear your path of any obstacles before you begin your journey—or before you continue it. Just as you wouldn't want to drive over debris on the road, and just as an airline pilot would never choose to fly through a storm if it could be avoided, clearing the way to Ultimate Recovery is an important first task if you want the best and fastest results from the approach detailed in this book. So before we get into the main topics, let's see if there is anything you can clear out of your way.

1. **Identify barriers you may have.** Problems such as diabetes, mental health issues, alcohol or substance abuse, or a serious communication or physical problem are examples of issues that may need to be managed so you are best able to take on the challenge of this Ultimate Recovery program. These are just examples. There are many things that may represent barriers to recovery.

   Take an honest look at your life circumstances. What significant barriers like the ones mentioned above might you have to creating and sustaining a healthy lifestyle? Notice I said "might." It's possible you don't have any. But this exercise can only help you, so please take the time to think through it carefully.

   Get a pen or pencil and spend a few minutes writing here about what you feel your most significant physical or mental health barrier(s) to living a healthy life might be. Write what it is and *why* you feel it may be a barrier for you.

2. **Talk with your doctor or other healthcare professional.** Before you go any further, make an appointment with your doctor or other trusted healthcare professional. Ask for their frank opinion concerning whether you have done everything possible to address the condition(s) you wrote about.

   Also ask them if they see any other barrier that might keep you from your goal of achieving and sustaining *best mental and physical health*. Take this book with you and write their response or ask them to write it for you in the space provided below.

3. **Ask for guidance regarding how to address the issue(s).** If you're already undergoing treatment for the issue you identified, or are planning to start, this treatment will become part of your Ultimate Recovery plan. Write the advice or treatment you have been given by a professional concerning the barrier you have identified. (If you need help writing, ask for help from someone you trust.)

It's up to you whether you will take any advice you receive. I strongly encourage you to consider doing so. If you're unsure, ask for another opinion from someone else who knows you well and you trust.

**Do your best to at least begin
to address any concerns above
before going further in this program.**

CHAPTER 2

CREATING CHOICE: OVERCOMING IMPULSIVENESS

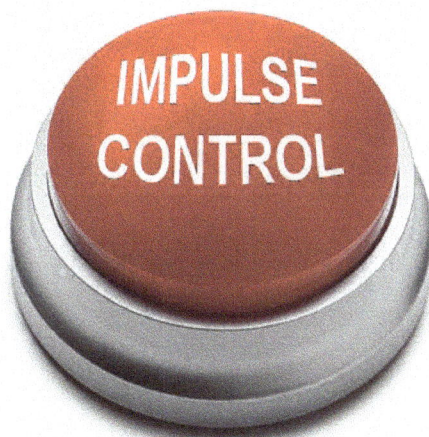

Definition of Impulsiveness:

"acting before thinking" or
"acting without thinking"

Impulsiveness is the enemy. If you've ever read comic books or seen movies based on them, you know that every superhero has his or her arch enemy. Lex Luthor was one of Superman's arch enemies. Old Lex was a supervillain with evil powers almost as formidable as Superman's. On a number of occasions he even beat Superman (temporarily, of course!).

Make no mistake about it—impulsiveness is the arch enemy of Ultimate Recovery. *That's because impulsiveness is the arch enemy of choice.* It is choice that is essential to achieving best mental and physical health.

When we have a goal, we need to do what must be done to achieve it. Ultimate Recovery is a goal, and the intentional lifestyle it requires demands that we make choices day in and day out to stick with the planned approach to life that is the subject of this book.

Two types of impulses. One type of impulse is to seek pleasure; the opposite type of impulse is to avoid unpleasantness. These two types of impulses exist from birth, and they are powerful. Neither involves any direct involvement of intellect or thought. Neither is the result of having made a choice. Impulses are inborn programs that operate automatically and rapidly and, until we learn to control them, before any thinking has a chance to occur.

These inborn impulses are useful up to a point. The impulses to eat and drink, for example, help ensure we don't starve to death or die of dehydration. Our impulse to avoid pain helps us learn to avoid dangerous things like touching a hot stove. But if we don't have the ability to stop and consider when it may be proper to override impulses, they can become monsters that ruin our life.

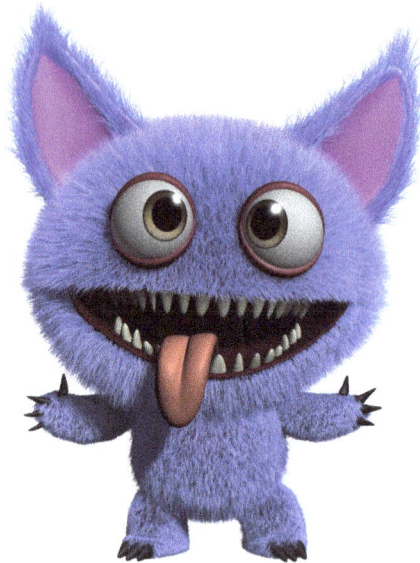

Impulses shouldn't govern us. We are blessed with intellect, which provides us with the ability to choose whether or not we will obey an impulse or override it. Impulses need to be overridden at times in order to accomplish things that require short-term pain in exchange for long-term gain. That's where the motto, "no pain, no gain," comes from.

With intellect, we can choose to deny the impulse to stay in bed, so we get up and get on with our day and move toward our goals. With intellect, we can choose to override our impulse to keep eating, so we go to the gym, exert effort, sweat, experience a bit of discomfort, and eventually reach our fitness goal. In order to finish high school, learn a sport, keep a job, raise a family, and/ or stay in shape, we must be able to override certain impulses. All these accomplishments involve putting up with some short-term unpleasantness to achieve the deep, long-lasting satisfaction that comes with them, satisfaction that impulses can never provide.

Impulses are always trying to steer us toward short-term pleasure and away from any discomfort. But as we've said, some of the most satisfying accomplishments might require us to ignore our impulses and endure short-term discomfort, inconvenience, and even pain in order to obtain something we want.

Without the ability to override impulses, humans would never have landed a man on the moon, found the cure for polio, or created beautiful paintings like the *Mona Lisa*. There would be no Olympic gold medals, and there would probably be none of the many marvels of science, art, and athletics we take for granted.

Bad choice or no choice? Many of the "bad choices" we make in life aren't really choices at all, just unthinking actions driven by impulse, by our desire for comfort or pleasure of some kind. If this sounds familiar, perhaps you have been described as impulsive sometime in your life.

If you think that to be impulsive means you lack intelligence, think again. Most people who earn the label "impulsive" have plenty of intelligence. They just haven't learned how to slow down and stop when necessary to give their intellect a chance to kick in and do its job in creating choice.

Impulse control requires brakes. If you have a car without adequate brakes, you walk, get a ride from someone, or take the bus until the brakes are repaired. It's just not possible to drive without brakes. There are times when we just have to slow down to maintain control and get where we're going.

When it comes to cars, we know this. But to control our impulses, slowing down is also required. Can you think of a time in the past when you could have avoided a predicament had you only slowed down or stopped to give yourself a chance to think?

When we were children, our ability to slow down, to reflect, choose, and follow a plan of action was undeveloped and simply not strong enough to overpower impulses. This is why, without adult guidance, children often select short-term gain and—without realizing it—long-term pain.

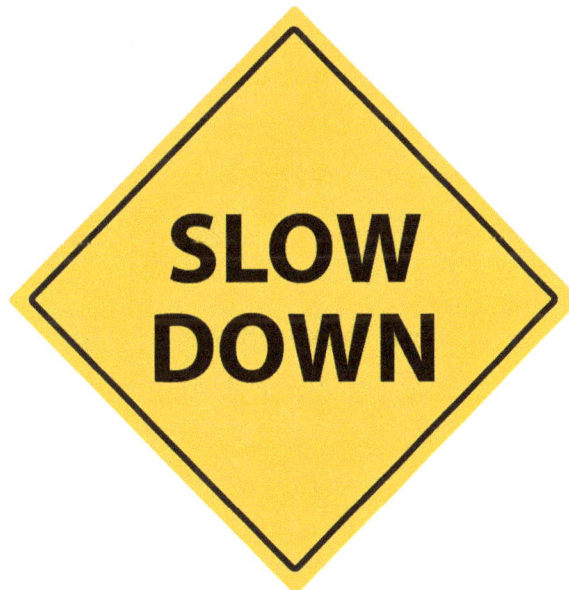

If you're having trouble thinking of a time that you failed to slow down and think as an adult, think back to when you were a child. Either will do for the following reflections.

Reflection: Failure to Apply the Brakes. Can you think of some mistake you made—when something unfortunate happened to you—because you just didn't think first?

Where and when did this failure occur?

_____

What happened (briefly)?

_____

_____

_____

Reflection: Success at Impulse Control. Can you think of something you accomplished, that made you proud, that involved following a plan and enduring some unpleasantness?

Where and when did this success occur?

_____

What happened (briefly)?

_____

_____

_____

Impulses never sleep and they act with the speed of light. By contrast, intellect needs time to function, and it requires periodic rest. If you're always doing things in a hurry, especially if you are neglecting your sleep, then you may be making it impossible for your intellect to have the time and energy it needs to control your impulses. Slowing down is among the most important things you can do to master impulse control.

Impulse control, intellect, and the executive functions. What we refer to as intellect arises from our frontal lobes, located right behind our forehead. Intellect includes four major functions: (1) being aware of what needs doing, (2) deciding what needs doing *now*, (3) creating a plan for doing those things that need doing, then (4) carrying out the plan. Collectively, these functions are known as the executive functions, and they are the means by which our intellect overrides and controls our impulses.

The frontal lobes
"the seat of Intellect"

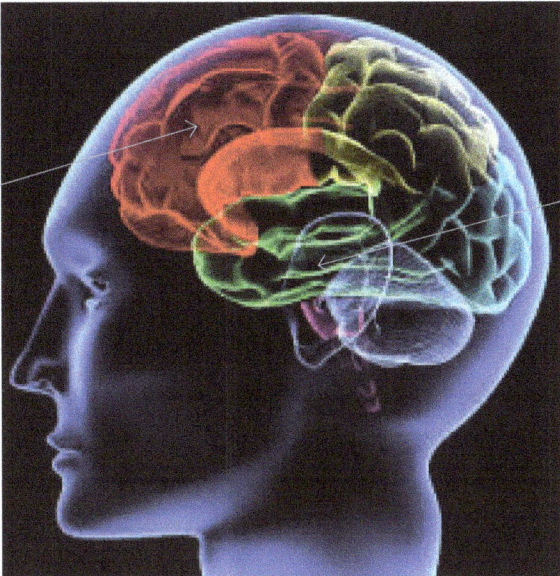

General region of the limbic system
"the seat of impulses"

The frontal area of our brain (see above left) is responsible for the executive functions. The area deeper in the brain that is responsible for impulses (see above right) exists in a dynamic tension with the executive functions throughout your lifetime. There's nothing wrong with pursuing pleasure and avoiding pain as long as doing so doesn't block your path to important goals, like achieving health and satisfaction. There are times when we simply must resist our impulses in order to accomplish something important to our well-being.

How our intellect becomes stronger than our impulses is explained by the story of the two wolves. This is an old Native American story used to teach children. The lesson of the story is as follows: "There are two wolves inside each of us, a good one and a bad one. The wolf that will win is the one you feed." This means when we allow our impulses (the "bad wolf") to control us, we feed them and make them stronger. By exercising our intellect (the "good wolf"), we feed it and make it stronger.

Which wolf do you feed, the intellectual or the impulsive one? Remember that we're born with powerful impulses. Our intellect, on the other hand, needs nurturance; it needs to be fed to gradually, over time, grow stronger than our impulses.

An Impulse-Driven Lifestyle Requires	An Intentional Lifestyle Based on the Choice to be Healthy Requires
Nothing is required. We're born with impulses that are preprogrammed and ready to go.	Practicing continuous awareness of your intention to be well.
	A plan to accomplish it.
Impulses are always awake, always ready to take control when your intellect is not leading.	Consistency in sticking with it.
	Recognizing when you've gotten away from your lifestyle plan despite your best intentions.
	Coming back to it, again and again.

The "cure" for impulsive living is to live with intention. When we take the time to reflect on and choose what we need and want most, create a plan to accomplish it, then follow our plan, we are living intentionally.

Perfection isn't necessary. *Practice is perfect.* That's another of our recovery mottos. It means that if you continue to return to practice whenever you get sidetracked, you'll get better.

Practice Is Perfect.

Beware a society that considers impulsiveness normal. "Normal" simply means what most people do. Acting normally can be a bad thing if most people you know live unhealthy lives.

Modern advertising is devoted to creating new and more effective ways for us to pursue pleasure. Alcohol/drugs, social media, video gaming, and pornography are among the biggest of what I call the lethal distractions. Shopping, gambling, partying, and web surfing are right up there as well. Most of these are OK in small amounts. They become *bad for us* when we are unable to resist them long enough to accomplish what it takes to create a lifestyle that leads to the mental and physical health we need, want, and deserve.

In modern society a lot of us are becoming addicted to various activities and substances, vastly strengthening our impulses. This tendency is so pervasive that some have said society itself is becoming dominated by impulse and has become sick as a result.

If you are an alcoholic or addict of any kind, you can probably count on getting feedback that what you are doing is unhealthy and destructive. But if your addiction is not something commonly recognized as an addiction, you may get nothing but encouragement from those who care about you.

For example, you go out and buy a pair of shoes you can't afford. Friends say, "Good for you! You need to treat yourself once in a while." Or you spend all day watching TV. Friends say, "Good for you! You need a day off now and then." Or you eat a pint of ice cream in a single sitting. Friends say, "Good for you! Nothing wrong with indulging yourself occasionally!" It's true that

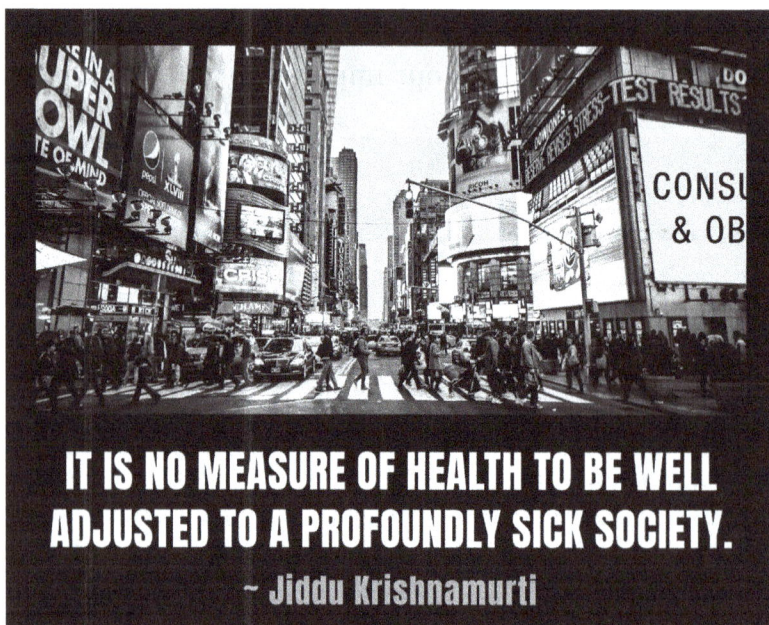

IT IS NO MEASURE OF HEALTH TO BE WELL ADJUSTED TO A PROFOUNDLY SICK SOCIETY.
~ Jiddu Krishnamurti

no one of these things will kill you. But repeatedly indulging your impulsive cravings will give you an impulsive, unhealthy lifestyle that eats away at whatever impulse control you have and slowly—or not so slowly—destroys your ability to pursue anything healthy.

Impulsiveness: an addiction with no name. There are those who don't engage in any one activity to excess but who instead flit from one to the other nearly nonstop. Those who alternate between distractions might never be thought of as an addict. But that's why I think of impulsiveness as the addiction with no name. It might be the most dangerous of all because, as we noted above, no one might notice so they might not ever think to say, "Stop—you are hurting yourself!"

Also as we noted above, you might even get encouragement from people who seem quite healthy but who themselves suffer from the addiction with no name. You might unwittingly have become a member of an impulsiveness club, where each member reinforces each other's dysfunction and no one realizes it.

Impulsiveness as a distraction from life. What are we really avoiding by distracting ourselves? Could it be Life itself? When we live according to impulse—as with any form of addiction—we may be simply avoiding Life *as it is*. Everyday life is mostly ordinary, normal, average. Exceptionally good or exceptionally bad days are, well, the exception!

But for the impulsive individual, ordinary, normal, and average may be intolerable. This is why some severely impulsive people will seesaw between feeling "really good"—on days they are able to fill with favorite distractions—or "really bad"—on days they are unable to do so.

A person in balance tends to experience their life more evenly. Most days are generally good, but do you notice? Most of us have shelter, food, clothing, and safety. But I believe many "normal" people today have lost the capacity to tolerate a good, normal, average, ordinary life. And if you can't tolerate normal, average, and ordinary, *you can't tolerate Life*. Then you're ripe for developing cravings and addictions.

How about you? Do encounters with normal, average, ordinary everyday experiences become triggers to seek a distraction? How long can you sit still and just relax? If your answer is "not very long," why not? What's the basis of that underlying itch you constantly need to scratch? A lot of this book is devoted to answering that very question.

Find and connect with people who share your ideas about health and recovery.

Again, keep in mind as we proceed that living impulsively has become normal for many in our society and perhaps for many of our friends and family. Living a life of excitement is often considered a sign of success, while living with a stable routine and a sense of purpose is often thought of as dull and boring. As a consequence, you may not get much encouragement from others to become healthy, stable, and purposeful. You may need to befriend those who share your values, who will support you, and who you can support. Be on the lookout for such people.

You will become what you practice.

Persistence. You will become what you practice. You are what you have practiced to this point in your life. Right now, this very day, you are becoming either more intentional and more physically and mentally healthy or more impulsive and less healthy depending on which style of living you have been practicing since arising this morning.

A recovery lifestyle will require change and change is difficult. "Persistence" means continuing to practice a healthy lifestyle despite difficulty. If you feel you lack persistence, be reassured that it too will develop over time if you just don't quit. You can't fail if you don't quit.

Be patient with yourself. Persist. Keep doing your best every day to practice the principles and practices outlined in this book. You're worth the effort. If you simply keep coming back to this program whenever you get off track, you'll keep moving forward. You can't fail if you don't quit.

Everyone experiences hopelessness and futility once in a while. Such feelings may indicate you are trying to accomplish something that is currently beyond your abilities. Perhaps you need to scale back your goals and expectations for a while until you become stronger. Your best effort will vary. Just don't quit.

If you find you have given in yet again to hours of aimless web surfing, eating, TV watching, video gaming, or what have you—if this is what is leading to your sense of futility and hopelessness, admit it to yourself. But be kind and gentle. Resolve to do better and remember that every time you come back to the plan outlined in this book, you are exercising impulse control. Each time you come back, you get stronger and better!

But if you just can't overcome impulsiveness despite everything written here, perhaps you have a real addiction. As I said above, I believe we're all addicted to something. But you might need to reflect on your situation with someone you trust or search for some type of professional help. If you're not sure, talk with your doctor or with a therapist. This too is persistence. Get the help you deserve.

You can't fail if you don't quit.

CHAPTER 3

GETTING UNSTUCK: DEALING WITH ANGER AND LOSS

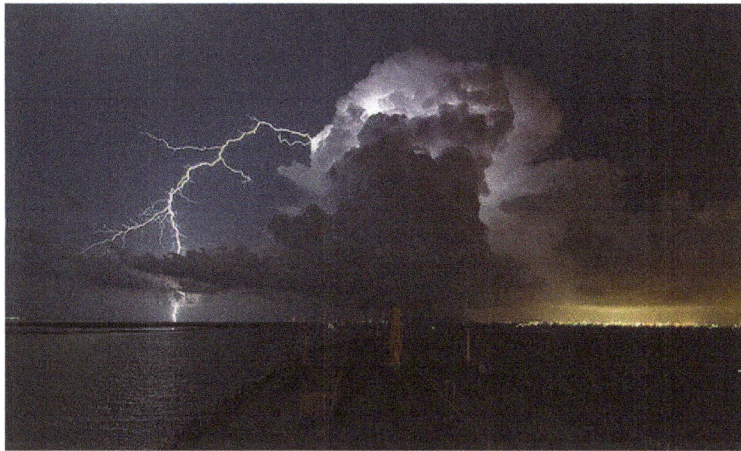

Where there is anger, there is pain.

What this chapter is for. The purpose of this chapter isn't to eliminate anger but to eliminate some of anger's more destructive effects. You'll still get angry at times, but with practice, you can learn to tame your anger and behave in a more conscious, intentional way, even in upsetting circumstances. So please read on.

Everyone gets angry. Everyone. Anger can be quiet or loud. It can pass quickly or linger for hours, days, or even years. It can be caused by something trivial, like not being able to find your socks. It can be caused by something major, such as being physically assaulted. We can feel angry on someone else's behalf, such as when we become angry when we see someone being neglected, taken advantage of, or abused.

Anger can serve a variety of purposes. Anger can give us the energy we need to defend ourselves or someone else physically or emotionally. It can help us snap back when we're feeling defeated. It might even provide a form of protection against the overwhelming emotion that follows a major event, like the death of a loved one.

But it's a double-edged sword. Although anger may serve a purpose in the short run, it can also result in damage to relationships, people, property, and our bodies, damage that lasts longer than and far outweighs any benefit. For example, it can prevent us from realizing we're over-reacting to trivial things (like those socks). It can cause others to avoid us and leave us isolated and bitter. It can create enemies when what we really need are allies. Perhaps most important, a reliance on anger as our go-to response prevents us from truly knowing and taking care of ourselves. That's because *anger is the lid on the pot; it's not what's cooking inside.* Experiencing and understanding deeper emotions require us to lift the lid and look inside the pot beneath the anger. That's where health, connection, and satisfaction are to be found.

What your body can teach you about anger. Your body can teach you a great deal about anger. When you get angry, you secrete adrenaline. Your heart and breathing rates increase. Your blood pressure rises. Your body goes into a ready state that has been called the fight or flight response. This means your body is preparing for a situation by either confronting it (fight) or running from it (flight). Our angry reaction indicates we are feeling threatened in some way.

Criticism, or even a judgmental glance, may trigger this response. In Dr. Herbert Benson's classic book, *The Relaxation Response* (coauthored with Miriam Z. Klipper), he suggests there may be dozens of triggers caused by dozens of small threats and followed by dozens of mini fight or flight responses in the course of a typical day. Most are subtle and barely noticeable. But our bodies are telling us there is something at risk, that we are being threatened in some way.

So the question is: "When we get angry, what is threatened? What are we trying to protect?" Asking ourselves this question can reveal what's really going on that anger is hiding from us.

Reflection: Identifying Anger. Take a minute to think about the following. Have you ever felt angry because of something someone did? Think about the last time you were *really* angry. Take a minute and get an actual situation in mind. Don't read on until you do this. Then briefly describe this situation below, including when and where it occurred.

Where and when did this occur?

What happened (briefly)?

Anger is a secondary emotion. Anger has been described as a secondary emotion. This means that anger is an emotion that is often a symptom of *other emotions*. So now think harder, *feel deeper*, beneath the anger you recalled above. Is something else there, another emotion?

What other feelings did you have *before* you became angry in the situation you described above? Think back and see if you can recall what you were feeling that day *right before you felt anger*. Write what you come up with below. Do this now before you read on.

Now see if you can recall a different instance of being angry. Take a minute and get a real situation that you experienced, including when and where it occurred. Write it below.

Where and when did this occur?

What happened (briefly)?

Now go deep once again and try to recall what other feelings you felt just before the anger came over you. Write down the words that describe these feelings below.

Compare your answers with others. Below are some of the feelings others have come up with when doing this exercise. Are any of these the same or similar to what you wrote above?

Frustration
Powerlessness
Embarrassment
Disappointment
Abandonment
Disrespect
Outrage
Shame
Guilt
Fear

Anger is often, if not always, the result of feelings like these that exist beneath the surface of our conscious mind. In other words, anger is a secondary response to these deeper, *primary emotions.*

Reflection: Uncovering the Roots of Anger. Refer to one of the situations you described above in which you were really angry with someone. Based on the situation you described earlier, try and answer the following questions.

What was being threatened?

_____

_____

What were you defending with your anger?

_____

_____

What was at stake? What did you fear losing?

_____

_____

Anger as a defense of self. Below are answers others have come up with to the questions above. Are any of these like what you wrote?

My <u>honesty</u> was under attack.

My <u>courage</u> was under attack.

My <u>intelligence</u> was under attack.

My <u>competence</u> was under attack.

My <u>worthiness</u> as a human being was under attack.

The word "my" is in each of the above statements. Anger may be our way of responding to a threat to *the image we have of who we are, the image we want others to have of us*. When our self is threatened in this way it can feel as if we are being physically threatened.

Self-doubt and shame. But if we are confident in ourselves, why does it matter what someone else thinks or says about us? Why does it trigger such anger? Why do we feel such hurt?

Many of us have had experiences in our life that have eliminated healthy self-doubt and replaced it with certainty, *certainty that we are <u>insufficient</u> in some way*. There is an emotion that underlies such feelings of inadequacy. That emotion is shame.

Shame is a powerful emotion we do our best to keep hidden, even from ourselves. We may be so successful that we don't even know it is there. That's another purpose of anger, to keep our shame hidden from us. In this case, anger is like a dragon we post at the entrance to a deep, dark cave in which we keep our shame hidden and buried.

Fear disguised. Anger is so very good at covering up our insecurities. Like that mythical dragon guarding a cave full of treasure, anger lies in wait beside our fear and insecurities, keeping them well hidden, out of view and out of reach. Like that dragon, anger is ready to breathe fire and destroy anyone or anything that tries to approach what we don't want anyone to see. In other words, *anger originates on the inside, not from anything outside of us*. It's simply not accurate to say that someone or something *made me angry*. Anger is in us. And it's always alert, always waiting to be challenged, like that dragon.

The anger dragon is prepared to fight to the death to protect a version of our self that we have crafted to conceal what we believe, down deep, to be the truth, namely, that we are insufficient, inadequate, even worthless. The anger dragon shows itself anytime we feel challenged or pushed beyond our limits. Anger can be a most effective way of feeling and acting strong while we protect a fragile self-image.

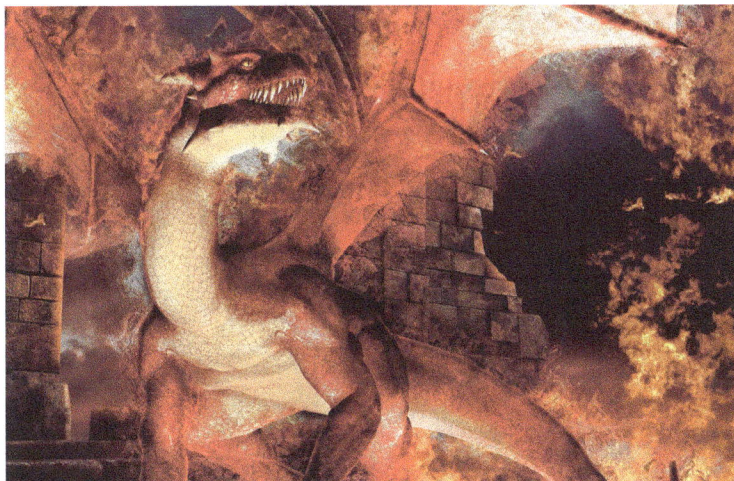

However, as long as we resort to anger to protect us, we ultimately keep ourselves from learning the truth: There is nothing wrong with us at all; the vulnerability, self-doubt, and even shame we might feel are emotions shared by many of us for surprisingly normal reasons. So as long as we resort to anger, we keep ourselves from ourselves. As long as we resort to anger, we also keep others away and keep ourselves isolated. And the longer we resort to anger, *the less brave and the more fearful of our real emotions we become.*

You may be denying having any feelings of fear or insecurity as you read this. But is it possible you have pushed these feelings to the back of a cave deep inside yourself? If you get angry easily, it's probable you've done just that.

But what you might be defending with your anger is your unhealthy, unhappy, *untruthful* beliefs about yourself; what you might be defending is your self-defeating and destructive behavior.

It's natural to feel vulnerable. Chances are, once again, that what underlies your anger is vulnerability and fear—or *fear of vulnerability.* Humans are highly vulnerable creatures who must depend on many factors over which we have limited control, such as air, food, water, and shelter. For these, we are dependent on having money. For money, we are dependent on a job, the government, or perhaps on our health benefits. We are at all times vulnerable to accident, sickness, old age, and, of course, death. So feeling vulnerable is the most natural emotion of all.

To be human means our exposure to being hurt and harmed from change and loss is constant. Given this, it's remarkable how well we manage to live our life as confidently as we do.

One of the ways we cope with vulnerability is by telling ourselves how powerful we are, by saying things like, "I can do anything I put my mind to." But somehow we know it's not true that we can do anything we put our mind to. We can't levitate above our chair, survive without air, or cheat death, for example. Human vulnerability is a fact of human life.

But we are so good at hiding our vulnerability from ourselves that when it is suddenly revealed by some sudden change or loss, it comes as a great shock to us, as a seismic tremor that shakes the foundations of our false sense of power and control. And because we are so good at hiding vulnerability from others (and they from us), when we suffer a loss, we may believe no one else can possibly understand how we feel.

Feeling your feelings makes you strong.

Feeling your feelings makes you strong. We bury hurtful feelings in the first place because they are unpleasant and painful. We may believe pain is harmful, so we must avoid it, push it away, lock it away, post our anger dragon to keep it safely hidden away, and then deny, deny, deny it is even there.

But why? Will feeling emotional pain really harm you? The answer is no; in fact, by allowing ourselves to identify, name, and feel our hurt, we can heal from it and become stronger than before. By allowing ourselves to become intimate with our emotions generally, we connect with ourselves and others. We learn that pain is just pain; suffering is just suffering. It comes; it goes. And it is the one thing we have in common with everyone else on the planet. Therefore, feeling your feelings is the basis of understanding and compassion.

Only once we allow ourselves to feel our deeper emotions can we learn that no matter how painful, our emotions cannot cause us harm. Feeling our feelings, both pleasant and unpleasant, is grounding ourselves in reality and making ourselves stronger to manage it.

The cost of continuing to deny feelings. Resistance to feeling our emotions is futile. They consume more and more of our energy in trying to resist them. Until we find a way to allow our emotions to surface, we may realize on some level how frozen in place we are, how stuck, how unable to move forward with our life we are. This is because emotions that are buried—especially hurtful ones—are emotions that can be all-consuming.

But this need not be the case. Healing from hurt is possible. Healing is necessary if best mental and physical health is your goal. You *deserve* to heal.

Futility is another word for hopelessness. Hopelessness can be the result of resisting our feelings of hurt and loss. If we don't develop the capacity to feel our feelings—including the yucky ones—they can become hopelessly stuck inside us.

Free the dragon. Remember the dragon? How miserable it is chained to the mouth of a cave, placed there by you as protection against the threat that someone will enter and discover what you've hidden there—all the hurt, the shame, and the other emotions you've buried there that you feel are unworthy, that you feel *make* you unworthy, and that *you are afraid to feel.*

But visiting the cave of hidden emotions and experiencing them once and for all is the path of healing. Only then will we experience healing and relief and come to realize that emotions felt are emotions freed. Allowing ourselves to feel painful feelings allows us to reconnect with the parts of ourselves we have cut off out of fear. *This reconnection frees us from the need for anger and removes a major barrier to Ultimate Recovery.*

Reconnecting with painful feelings makes you strong.

Once we have gained the courage to feel, we can finally set the anger dragon free, because it is no longer needed to protect us. And when we no longer fear our vulnerable and fearful feelings, it is natural for us to no longer fear that others will discover we have them. Then we can become stronger, more understanding, and more compassionate.

Of course, this is all easier said than done. But do you think you might be ready to liberate your anger dragon? Need help? All you have to do is ask, starting with the person in the mirror.

Loss: The mother of all hurts. Beyond insult, beyond injury, beyond the many types of pain we humans experience, there is loss. Loss represents a permanent inability to return to things as they were. Loss leaves no option but to move on to a life that will be different in some way from the one that existed before experiencing the loss.

The loss of a job, of a relationship or loved one, losses of body function, the loss of youth and health—these are examples that almost everyone has experienced or will experience in their lifetime. Loss is very simply a part of everyone's life. This is why loss is another of the marks of existence that everyone bears.

A brain injury may create loss on a physical, cognitive, emotional, and spiritual level. Your body may be different. You mind may be different. Your personality may be different. Your relationships may be different. Your self-image may be different. Chances are your finances are significantly changed. Friends and family relationships have likely shifted. Some relationships may have ended. The sense of loss can be mild or profound.

But remember that loss isn't unique to you. Loss is very simply part of what it means to be human. Everyone experiences loss.

Grief. We derive part or all of our sense of who we are from what we attach to. We can be attached to things, people, beliefs, memories, and/or dreams. Loss of any of these can make us feel the intense sense of loss we call grief. Grief is the emotional acknowledgment that we have lost something we loved.

But people respond to loss on their own timetable. Some of us allow ourselves to feel and to grieve after a loss. Others bottle up feelings, put off grief, bury it in that cave, post the dragon, and deny the loss. Similar to anger and the feelings underlying it, trying to bury our grief can become harmful to our mental and physical health.

There may be good reasons to deny loss and put off grieving at first. Perhaps if we allowed feelings of loss to surface right away, we would become too overwhelmed to function. Burying feelings may be the only option until some time has passed. Sometimes it takes months or even years before a person can afford to feel the full impact of what they have been through and begin to grieve.

But grieving, which is feeling the feelings associated with loss, is a healthy, essential process. It ultimately results in healing and being able to move beyond our losses. Each person's readiness to actively grieve will occur on a different schedule. There is no hard and fast rule concerning how much time it takes to be able to grieve and no hard and fast rule concerning how long the grieving process itself will take once it begins.

What is important to understand, wherever you're at, is that just as it is possible to become stuck in anger, it is possible to become stuck in grief or in the avoidance of it.

Is denial harmful? Probably not, if you're just not ready to experience your loss. But periodically it may be good to check in and consider whether you are ready to allow yourself to feel the sadness, hurt, and other emotions that go along with a significant loss. There's a part of you that ultimately needs to be heard and felt in order to regain health and wholeness.

Is there anything to be gained by feeling the pain of loss? Yes. As long as you're ready to grieve, relief is one of the benefits of active grieving. Another is freeing the emotional energy we were expending to hold off our grief. The pain of loss is actually a measure of how much our life matters to us. So another benefit of healthy grieving is regaining your appreciation for Life and your capacity to live Life to the fullest.

Therefore, while feeling loss is painful, it is also the means by which we release that pain, the method by which we relieve ourselves of the weight our loss burdens us with, and the path along which we can begin to move toward self-acceptance, gratitude, wholeness, compassion, and health.

Getting unstuck: Identify, name, feel, and share. Identify what you're feeling and name those emotions, allow yourself to really feel these emotions, and share them with someone you trust. This is a very powerful formula for weakening the grip of anger and loss on your life and strengthening relationships.

But identifying feelings, being clear enough about them to be able to name them, and developing the confidence to feel and share them may require professional guidance. If you believe you may be stuck in anger or grief, have you mentioned this to a therapist? If you don't have a therapist, will you consider getting one? If you quickly answered "no" just now, was your no a conscious, well-considered response or was it a reflexive, impulsive response?

You *deserve* recovery. You *deserve* best mental and physical health. Remind yourself of this often. And remind yourself that you cannot fail to achieve best mental and physical health if you are willing to do what it takes and never quit. If professional help *might* help you heal, why not give it a try?

Perhaps you're ready to take a leap of faith. If you agree you deserve recovery, don't rule out anything that might help you achieve it, including professional help. You may be very surprised at how good you feel as you heal emotionally. And that, after all, is the point of this book.

It may help to realize that therapists are acutely aware they too have anger and hurt, and most will admit they have used denial at times to deal with their feelings. We are all in the same boat when it comes to how to attempt to deal with vulnerability and hurt.

Summary. We've covered a lot in this chapter on a challenging subject. Here are the main ideas:

- Anger is a secondary emotion. Feelings of powerlessness, vulnerability, loss, and other hurtful emotions often trigger it.

- In the short run, anger may serve a purpose by giving us the energy to survive a big blow to our image of our self.

- In the long run, anger is a loser as a coping strategy. It alienates people in our life and can prevent us from knowing ourselves and providing for our deepest emotional needs.

- It's hard to allow ourselves to feel deeper feelings, especially vulnerability and fear, because we fear being consumed by them or because we fear that displaying them will make us appear weak to others.

- Fear of feeling vulnerability and fear is the deepest obstacle to experiencing and sharing our emotions. Giving in to fear tends to make it worse over time.

- Feeling and sharing our feelings of vulnerability are the only ways to free ourselves from fear of them and the only way to realize how common these feelings are.

- Sharing deep feelings of vulnerability and fear with someone who has hurt or frightened us, who we otherwise trust, can be a powerful way to build a stronger relationship.

- Facing and sharing deep feelings weaken our tendency to use anger as a coping mechanism.

- Hopelessness is a symptom of our futile efforts of continuing to deny vulnerability and loss. It takes more and more energy over time to keep them buried.

- Feeling is a primary element of Ultimate Recovery.

Let's stop and take a breath. This chapter has attempted to discuss some of the most difficult subjects associated with recovery and best mental and physical health. If you are feeling a bit drained after reading it, it is because you allowed yourself to feel. That's very good! As I said in the very beginning of the book, *feeling is what recovery is made of.*

Take a deep breath.
It's just a bad day,
not a bad life.

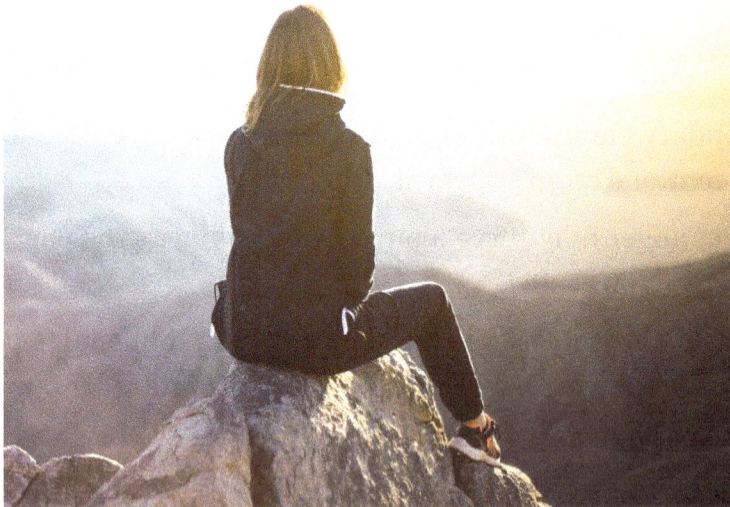

FOUNDATIONS OF ULTIMATE RECOVERY

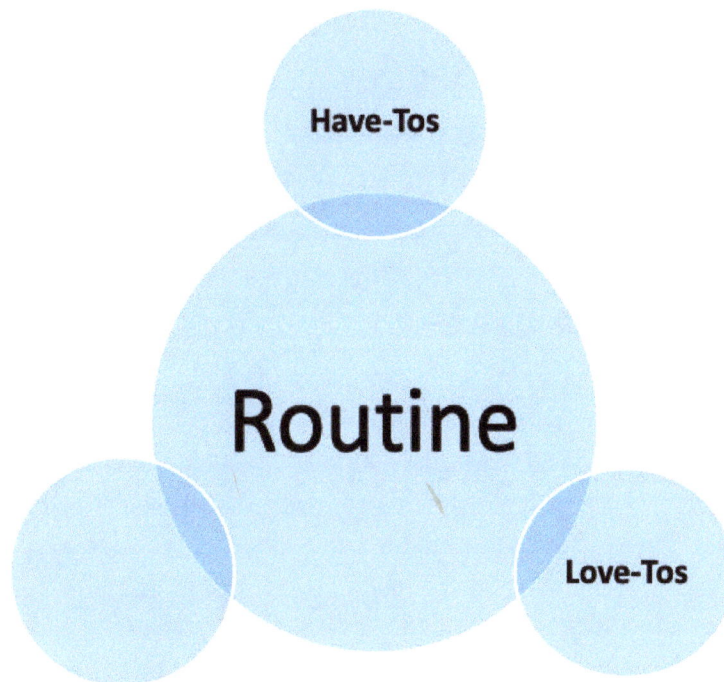

Have-Tos

Routine

Love-Tos

CHAPTER 4

LIVING INTENTIONALLY

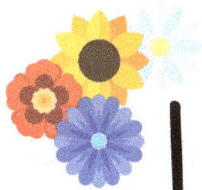

LIVE YOUR LIFE.
on purpose.

The wake-up call. No one is ever the same after a major life event. Some of the changes may be obvious, some less so. Some may not be obvious to you but very obvious to others. In any case, here is one you may well have overlooked: Major life events, especially those that involve a brush with death, tend to provide us with an essential realization or wake-up call.

Such an event can make us realize that Life is precious, that Life never stays the same, that Life itself is limited, and that someday it will be over. Most survivors I have worked with over the years admit that they did not have this awakening until after their injury. Before being injured, most admitted they said things like, "It's just another day," "There's always tomorrow," and "same old, same old." But because most survivors have had a brush with death, they no longer feel that way.

If that is true for you, then in a very real way *your injury didn't just take from you—it gave you something as well: a sense of urgency,* an urgency to make up for lost time. This new urgency is likely to be uncomfortable. At times, or perhaps all the time now, it might be downright painful.

Pain is *another* 'mark of existence'. This mark is the pain of realizing the truth about Life, that there is something at stake, namely, your whole life! When we begin to realize that Life is precious and our time on Earth is limited, we may begin to question how we have been living and begin to ask, *How am I supposed to live? What constitutes a good life?*

If you look closely at the faces of others, you will see that many people—*perhaps most people*—bear this mark, whether they are rich or poor, financially successful or struggling, alone or surrounded by friends. If you look closely enough at just about anyone, with or without a brain injury, you will see some of the self-doubt and anxiety that you may be feeling right now.

There are so many paths. Which to take?

A very good start. If you can identify with at least some of this, you are off to a very good start. You are realizing that how you approach Life and living matters. Despite the fact that you are unsure how to proceed, an opportunity is opening for you to make the most of the rest of your life.

We think of doubt as bad, but doubt has gotten a bad rap. Doubt must precede wisdom. It is only when we doubt that we stop and reflect. If we stop long enough to really see and feel what is going on, we can decide what we *can* do. After a bit longer we can decide what we *should* do. Finally, with a bit more stillness and reflection, we can decide what we *will* do.

Thus, our journey begins.

Don't expect others to understand what you are feeling. Others you know may not have this realization. They may not treat this minute, this day, this week, this month, this life, as if it matters, and so they may feel free to waste time, energy, talents, resources, and relationships. Try not to be so influenced by what these people say or do.

As a result of believing there will always be another tomorrow, many of us fail to ever appreciate or truly live our life. Instead, we waste time because we simply never feel the urgency you may be feeling right now. This is understandable because we live in a society that often denies reality, *especially the reality that Life is short and time is precious.*

Until the wake-up call, as I said above, you may have felt that each day was pretty much the same and today didn't matter that much. But the wake-up call is about realizing tomorrow is promised to no one, and the only thing you can count on is what is right here, right now. Thus, it is what you do right here, right now that matters.

Trust yourself that if you commit to trying what is written in the pages that follow, you will know whether or not the ideas and suggestions are right for you. Let your sense of urgency propel you forward to make changes that will bring you the best possible mental and physical health.

And always remember that you *so* deserve it.

Decisions, decisions. So how will you respond to this wake-up call to Life? How will you proceed from here? You have several choices. One we'll call the Bucket List Approach, and another we'll call the Smell the Roses Approach. Let's compare them.

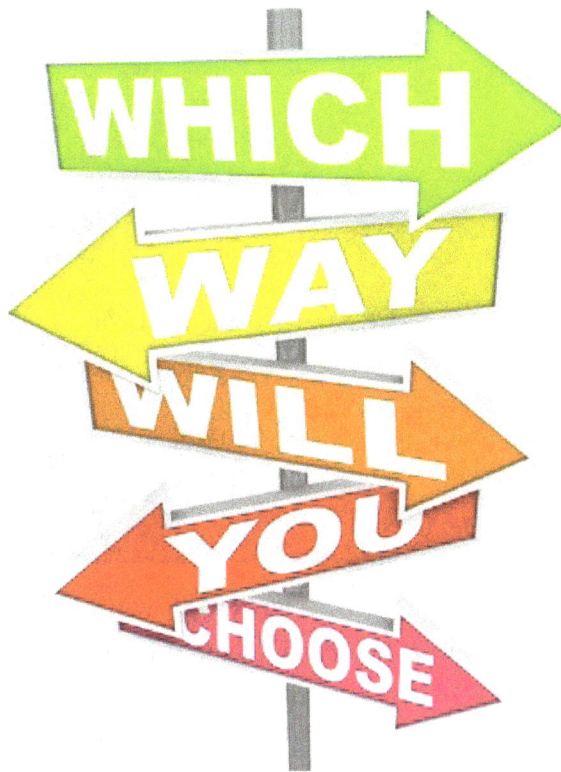

1. **The Bucket-List Approach.** This approach is characterized by exhortations of, "Hurry up! "Get going! Make your bucket list and cram in as much as possible before you kick the bucket!" This approach is about making up for lost time in the time you have left on the planet. It's a concept that's been around for eons but got more popular after the movie of the same name.

   This is certainly an understandable response to that sense of urgency we talked about, but it may also fuel a craving for excitement and living your life at a frantic pace that cause you to overlook and leave behind some great aspects of your life, including people you love and who love you.

   In its most extreme version, the Bucket List Approach is characterized by a desperate attempt to escape anything negative—any loss, hurt, limit, restriction, or discomfort of any kind—in an attempt to "be free."

   As a result, this approach can easily lead to addictions of all kinds: drugs, alcohol, compulsive shopping, eating, sex, gambling, work, or just plain busy-ness. Over time, more and more stimulation may be needed for less and less enjoyment. This can lead to a downward spiral into chronic anger, depression, isolation, or even premature death.

Let's look at another approach.

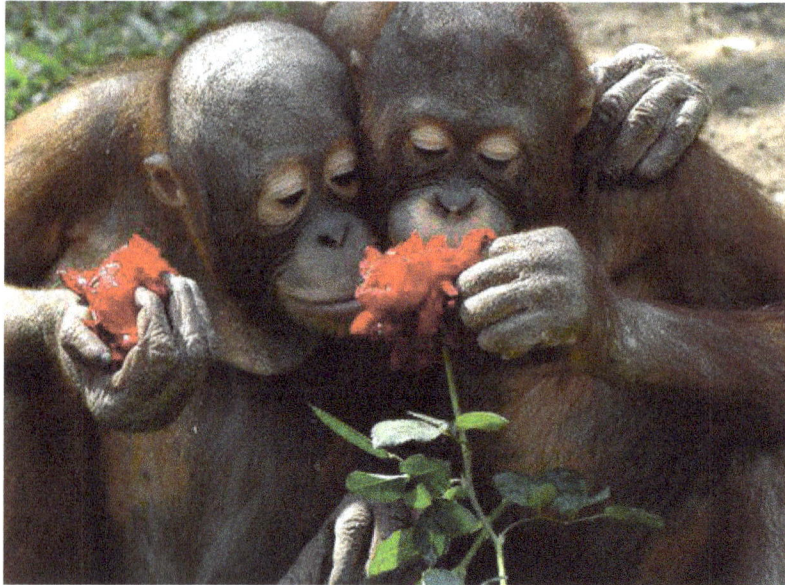

2. **Smell the Roses Approach.** This one says, "Slow down! What's your rush? Take it easy. Look around you and smell the roses! Learn to appreciate your life and all the little things and all the people you are lucky enough to have in it." At first, this may sound healthier than the Bucket List Approach, but again, if this approach is carried to an extreme, it can be just as big a problem as trying to empty your bucket. It can lead to not just slowing down but becoming self-preoccupied and becoming a couch potato and neglecting relationships, opportunities, and talents.

3. **Blended Approach.** Luckily, there is a third choice, a blending of the first two choices, a path that runs between the two extremes of "thrillin" (Bucket List) and "chillin" (Smell the Roses).

We will refer to this middle way as the Intentional Living Approach.

intentional

in · ten · tion · al
Adjective: Done on purpose; deliberate.

Intentional Living Approach. We live our life either consciously with specific goals in mind and a plan for achieving them, or we live more or less unconsciously according to impulse and habits we have acquired throughout our lifetime—impulses that may lead in an unhealthy direction and habits, if they lack clear intention, that lead in no particular direction at all.

Intentional Living is based on being clear about what you want and what you need then managing your life in order to achieve it. This book is about how to create a life based on the conscious intention to achieve best mental and physical health. It is an approach that involves a way of life not a one-time achievement. It is an approach that epitomizes what I call Ultimate Recovery.

If what you've been doing until now is satisfying and fulfilling for you, there's no reason to change. But if a lifestyle designed to maximize your best mental and physical health seems like the right way to approach your recovery, all you need to do is keep reading and gradually implement the practices presented in this book.

Simple and effective. This book outlines an approach that is pretty simple. It begins with choosing to try your best to *routinely* do three things: things that have to be done, things you love doing, and things that directly promote mental and physical health—whether or not you like them—because they work! It's an approach that cannot fail if you do not quit.

You can't fail if you don't quit.

A PATHWAY TO INTENTIONAL LIVING

A MAJOR LIFE-CHANGING EVENT

Especially the catastrophe of a brain injury, severe physical injury or illness, death of a loved one

↓

THE WAKE-UP CALL

"Life is short; time is precious; let me get busy living!"

↓

GETTING SERIOUS

Commit to achieve and sustain health as a priority, foundational goal.

↓

REFLECTING ON BARRIERS TO RECOVERY & LEARNING TO OVERCOME THEM

What serious health challenges have you yet to manage? Any chronic health problems—such as depression, diabetes, bipolar disorder, addiction, or a communication or physical impairment—can be a barrier to Ultimate Recovery. Commit to meeting with your doctor or a therapist to reduce such barriers.

↓

LIFESTYLE MANAGEMENT

Learn and practice—lifelong—the 7 Ultimate Recovery Practices that will allow you to achieve and sustain best mental and physical health.

Intentional living is about choosing, again and again, to create a lifestyle that promotes best mental and physical health.

CHAPTER 5

WHAT IS "BEST MENTAL AND PHYSICAL HEALTH"?

Best versus perfect. In my day-to-day life, some days are better than others. There are many factors that influence how I feel, even moment to moment, like how much sleep I got last night, the weather, how my wife and family are doing, what's going on in the world, how things are going for me financially, and, of course, my health. Each of these may affect the others in some way. Any change in one could change everything. And something is always changing. So each day, each hour, each moment of my life might fluctuate. You've probably noticed this.

So my best will also fluctuate. My best will be better on some days than others. And so will yours. That's real. Perfect consistency is not real. Perfect consistency isn't possible and isn't necessary to achieve Ultimate Recovery. What a relief! Let's move on.

Doing the best to do your best. All that is necessary to achieve Ultimate Recovery is to do your best to do your best, the best you are capable of right now. That will be enough. That will be *plenty*. If you do your best to return to the principles and practices contained in this book, you'll see results. Remember: You can't fail if you don't quit. Keep reminding yourself of that—it's true.

Best mental and physical health—breaking it down. The Ultimate Recovery lifestyle is a formula for best mental and physical health, and it can be grouped into the following activities. Each will be discussed in the coming chapters. Best mental and physical health is:

Making your best commitment to being healthy today. Remind yourself of your commitment frequently. Reaffirm it every day. You may want to post a sign on your refrigerator or wear some piece of jewelry that reminds you of your commitment to yourself. Most of us need some reminder to help us stay in touch with what matters most to us, so we aren't so easily distracted by the complexities of our life.

Making your best effort to be organized in your approach to creating a healthy lifestyle. It's really not hard. Routine is the subject of Chapter 7, and it will come up a lot. We'll refer to routine as the mother of recovery.

Making your best effort to maintain your strength, mobility, and endurance. You may have a lot of these or next to none. You may be able to improve a lot or just a little. Everyone is different. But whatever you have, don't take it for granted. Do the best you can to maintain what you have and increase it if you can. We'll talk about how in the chapter on the Practice of Fitness.

Making your best effort to be realistic in your expectations of yourself and your life. Being realistic is hard. Even knowing what is and isn't realistic can be tough in this modern world that promotes a video game version of life. We'll talk about this in some depth in the chapter on the Practice of Realism.

Making your best effort to be self-accepting. Judgement, ridicule, abuse: Many of us have experienced these things, sometimes at our own hands. The chapter on The Practice of Self-Acceptance will help you learn how to become your own best friend.

Making your best effort to take notice of and be grateful for all you have. We all notice what's wrong. That's quite natural. A lot of what we call negativity is actually built into the human brain's basic programming. But you can train yourself to notice the many good things that are always there, which you are probably overlooking. We'll cover this in the chapter on the Practice of Gratitude.

Making your best effort to be clear about what matters to you. We all pretend to be a lot clearer about things than we actually are. Clarity of mind is the result of a straightforward practice we'll cover in the chapter on the Practice of Clarity.

Making your best effort to maintain your peace of mind, which we'll call serenity. If we let it, Life will keep us spinning faster and faster until our head feels like it's about to explode. It's not that hard to reverse this and begin to experience deep calm and groundedness. That's the subject of the chapter on the Practice of Serenity.

Making your best effort to show up for your life, not just physically but also mentally. Showing up requires leaning into the activities that make up your day and the social interactions that make your relationships. Instead of showing up, our mind tends to take us away, often to the past or the future where we spend a lot of time regretting or worrying. This is not only distressing but robs us of the experience of our actual life and of the vitality to live it. the Practice of Presence chapter describes a powerful technique for living your real life with dignity and ease.

And remember: You can't fail if _____ _____ _____.
Nice. You're on the path to Ultimate Recovery!

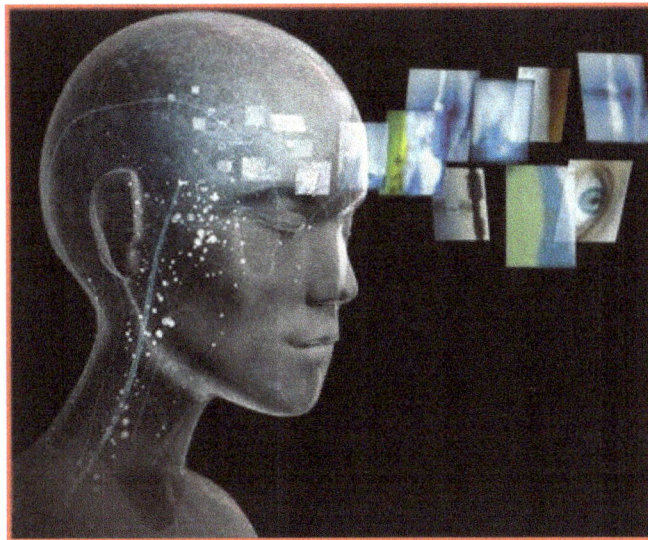

CHAPTER 6

TURN OFF YOUR AUTOPILOT: BECOME MORE CONSCIOUS

Review. Ultimate Recovery begins with understanding that Life is unpredictable, uncontrollable, ever-changing. The fact that you had an injury is one example of this. But there are countless instances of unwanted changes that occur in everyone's lives, changes we are powerless to do anything to prevent. And although we can't control many of the circumstances of our life, we often can control *how we live with those circumstances*.

How a person lives is what we call lifestyle. An Ultimate Recovery lifestyle is a particular way of life, the result of an intention to be mentally and physically healthy and therefore to live according to a routine that includes and organizes three main life activities: things we *have* to do, things we *love* to do, and the *7 Recovery Practices*. In addition to providing a pathway to recovery from brain injury, we've also noted that the Ultimate Recovery lifestyle is among the surest ways to recover from any future setback Life may have in store for us.

The Ultimate Recovery lifestyle will very likely be new and quite different than any way you have lived before. It will therefore require a high level of awareness or consciousness so you can consistently choose to practice the new, healthy patterns of living rather than giving in to old, unconscious habits.

In earlier chapters we talked about how impulses and anger can interfere with our ability to make choices and keep us stuck in old ways of responding. But impulses and anger are only two interferences to making conscious, thoughtful choices. Let's look at a few others.

Conditioned behaviors. Conditioning isn't something we're born with like impulses. Conditioned behaviors are learned through experience. It's good we don't have to make a conscious choice each time we cook whether or not to put our hand on a hot burner. We don't have to because everyone of us has probably been conditioned to keep our hands away from intense heat as a result of having been burned once in the past.

Conditioning is learning that's so powerful it causes us to act automatically without thinking, without having to make a decision. I recall running down a hill when I was about five years old. I tripped, and when I put my hands out to break my fall, my left palm landed on a shard of glass from a broken bottle. It made a gash that bled all over. I still have the scar. I was shocked by the pain and blood. I was lucky my dad—a WWII corpsman—was with me to bandage me right up with a handkerchief he always carried. As a result of this experience, I was conditioned to be on the lookout for tripping hazards.

On another occasion I was pounding a nail and I hit my thumb—hard! As a result of the incredible pain experienced that one time, I was conditioned to be a lot more careful when I use a hammer. I slow down and take careful aim. I don't have to remember to do this. I have become conditioned to do it automatically.

Any experience that provides a powerful reward or a powerful punishment can result in automatic, conditioned behavior patterns.

Have you ever been conditioned by some powerful positive or negative experience? Describe it briefly here:

_____

_____

_____

_____

Habits. As children we are taught how to act around others. It may require that the lessons be repeated before they are fully learned, but if our parents, teachers, or other caregivers are patient and persistent, we eventually master this kind of learning until the behavior becomes an unconscious habit. We accumulate a lot of habits from peers as well, especially as teenagers.

At that stage peers become powerful influences, and we model ourselves after the behaviors of those we look up to or just to fit in and be accepted.

When someone puts out their hand and says, "Hi, my name is Bob," most people will respond by extending their own hand, shaking Bob's hand, and introducing themselves. This is behavior we have learned through repetition to perform automatically. Chances are you won't remember Bob's name in a minute or two due to the fact you were acting without thinking and probably not listening when he said his name.

Can you think of an example of a habit you have that you now perform automatically? Write about it briefly here:

_____

_____

_____

More examples of behavior performed on autopilot. These behaviors also do not involve decision-making. Based on the above descriptions, check the type of behavior that best describes the example and give your reason.

- Many of us have some dread of going to the dentist. Just making an appointment may elicit a shiver down our spine as the recollection of pain or discomfort is recalled at the mere mention of the word "dentist." This is an example of
  __ an impulse __ conditioning __ a habit because:

_____

_____

- If you have had a negative experience with a person identified with a particular political, racial, or religious group, you might have an automatic negative response later to another person you met who is a member of the same group, even though you know nothing else about them. This is an example of
  __ an impulse __ conditioning __ a habit because:

_____

_____

Comment: This is the basis of prejudice and hatred, and it can be passed on from generation to generation, assuring the continuation of social discord and injustice.

- BMW is a popular car. We see advertising where cool, attractive, well-dressed people are driving and getting in and out of BMWs. We see commercials on TV where the cars whip around turns effortlessly. We know they cost a lot and are associated with prestige and success. Many of us see such cars and feel an attraction to them. This is an example of
  __ an impulse __ conditioning __ a habit because:

Comment: This is the whole point of advertising, to program us to have strong, positive, and automatic associations with a product—in this case, a car. Such advertising can create a need to possess status symbols in order to feel worthwhile and acceptable. Most of us have fallen prey to such advertising, maybe not concerning cars, but what about the handbag, sunglasses, shoes, etc., that you just have to have? Advertising is an extremely well-thought-out, extremely effective form of programming.

- When I first met Bob a week ago, he seemed cold and aloof. Although I smiled and responded warmly to him, he barely looked up. He shook my hand limply. I had a negative reaction. Here he comes again, and I'm having a similar reaction. My first impression of him a week ago programmed me. I walked the other way trying to avoid contact with him today. This is an example of
  __ an impulse __ conditioning __ a habit because:

Comment: If I happen to work with Bob, this programming may prevent me from having a good relationship with him. And this kind of programming may keep me from recognizing that Bob is another human being, a mixture of positive and negative traits, just like me. The problem is the negative first impression inclines me to not give him any more chances—too bad for him and for me.

- I am listening to a commercial on the radio about a well-known beer. I have seen many commercials during the Super Bowl with lots of attractive people having fun drinking this beer. When I hear a radio commercial later, the TV images and the fun feelings they produced during the Super Bowl return to me. Maybe I'll go get a beer after work. This is an example of _an impulse _conditioning _a habit because:

Comment: This programming can be downright disastrous if I suffer from alcoholism and it causes me to drink again. And again, advertising is all about programming us so we consume products of all kinds. Advertising works! Our best defense is to become conscious of our thoughts, feelings, and behaviors so we can exert some control over them.

- I take an adult education class with a woman named Tara. She is always the first to raise her hand to answer the teacher's questions. Boy, does she bug me! Who is she trying to impress? Why doesn't she keep quiet and let the rest of us talk? This is an example of _an impulse _conditioning _a habit because:

Comment: Without realizing it, I am responding to programming from long ago, from when I was in elementary school. There were kids like Tara in my class back then. They made fun of me. I felt embarrassed and ashamed. I have been programmed to feel negatively whenever I am around anyone who reminds me of those days.

Many of us have a ton of this old programming. We encounter people who remind us of other people in our past. *Most of the time the association with someone else is unconscious.* If the people we are reminded of are people we dislike, we judge the person in front of us negatively. If we are unconscious of what is going on, we can deny ourselves relationships that might turn out to be extraordinary ones given a chance. A chance at what? To prove they are humans like us—a mixture of positive and negative. What if we could accept that everyone truly is a combination of positive and negative? Might it help us accept that we too are this mixture, and might that allow us to more readily accept ourselves?

- I walked into a store and had trouble finding what I was looking for. I stopped a salesperson to ask a question. I politely said, "Excuse me, may I ask you a question?" The salesperson looked up blankly, gave out a little sigh, and said, irritably, "Yeah?"

I immediately felt a tension in my stomach and started to feel anger. This is an example of __ an impulse __ conditioning __ a habit because:

_____

_____

Comment: If you were conscious of your internal reaction and later revisited this experience, you might realize you felt embarrassed and disrespected by the salesperson's reaction. The anger you started to feel was actually an unconscious, programmed effort to cover up the vulnerability you were feeling. You might realize that just about any time you get angry, it is because you are being made to feel vulnerable. You could learn in this way to appreciate how sensitive we humans are and that anger is often an indication of hurt.

Reflection: How Conscious Are You? Are you conscious enough of the time *to choose your behavior* enough of the time *to develop a new Ultimate Recovery lifestyle?* Or *are you mostly on autopilot?*

Write down a time that you *chose* your behavior. In other words, you stopped, considered, and consciously decided to act the way you acted. Describe it briefly below.

_____

_____

_____

Now try to determine how much of your behavior each day you consciously choose. How much of what you do is controlled by you versus how much is the result of impulses, conditioning, and habits? For most of us, almost everything we do is the result of one of these. This is another way of saying we hardly ever think before we act! We almost always act automatically as a result of our impulses, conditioning, and habits.

If our goal is to choose to live in a new, more healthy way, we will need to choose our behavior.

Try rating your level of conscious behavior in an average 24-hour period by circling the rating below you think is most accurate. Before you complete your rating, remember that *everything you do is a behavior.* Tossing and turning during sleep, sneezing, scratching, frowning, smiling, washing the dishes, walking the dog, shopping, and carrying on a conversation—*we're never not behaving.*

Self-Rating

On a scale of 1 to 10, where 1 is Automatic, Unconscious, Reflexive and 10 is Intentional, Conscious, Thoughtful, circle the number below that represents your behavior most of the time:

AUTOMATIC									INTENTIONAL
UNCONSCIOUS									CONSCIOUS
REFLEXIVE									THOUGHTFUL

1   2   3   4   5   6   7   8   9   10

I personally rate myself a 4 on this scale. I'm trying to get to around a 5 or 6, so I can be more mindful of what I am doing during the day and make choices consistent with my own Ultimate Recovery plan. I don't want to have to think about *everything* (I don't want to be a 10). I do want to become more conscious, more aware of myself, and to slow down a bit so I can more easily stop and think whenever it's called for.

I feel like I need a lot of practice. Good thing I have the rest of my life. And good thing I know I can't fail if I don't quit.

How about you?

Are you conscious enough of the time to *choose your behavior* enough of the time to *develop a new, Ultimate Recovery lifestyle?* Or are you mostly on autopilot?

Exercise: Turning Off Your Autopilot. As we have seen above, automatic behavior can be positive or negative depending on the situation. The problem is, it can only be evaluated *after* you have done what the programming demanded. If the result was positive, then no problem. But if the result was negative, it may be impossible to undo what was done.

But what if you were able to detect automatic behavior and stop it so you could decide whether or not to proceed? In other words, what if you were able to turn off your autopilot? Is it possible? Let's find out.

In this exercise I want you to focus on automatic behaviors that involve negative reactions, as they (a) may be easier to detect than others, and (b) they have the potential to create bigger problems.

Let's see how many automatic responses you can catch as they are happening or just before they happen. Try to catch yourself acting on autopilot. Any number of things can trigger a negative automatic behavior. You may be triggered by someone or something that someone did or said.

Try to detect at least two such situations before moving on to the next chapter.

Tip: Negative programming might be accompanied by a warning. You could feel a contraction somewhere in your body—your stomach, back, neck, face, arms, or legs, etc. As soon as you sense any physical reaction, hit the brakes—in other words, *stop* and take notice if you can. That means to actually stop moving and stop talking for at least a second. And then take a conscious breath before you continue.

1. **First Occurrence.** Write below something that triggered you today. (Note: It may be something that actually happened or something you just expected would happen.)

_____

_____

_____

Did you have a physical sensation at the time? What did you feel? Where did you feel it?

_____

_____

_____

Were you able to apply the brakes? Were you able to stop moving and stop talking momentarily? _Yes _No

If you stopped, how did that feel?

_____

_____

What happened after you started moving again? Was it different, do you think, than what would have happened if you hadn't stopped? In what way?

_____

_____

_____

2. **Second Occurrence.** Write below something that triggered you today. (Note: It might be something that actually happened or something you just expected would happen.)

_____

_____

_____

Did you have a physical sensation at the time? What did you feel? Where did you feel it?

_____

_____

_____

Were you able to apply the brakes? Were you able to stop moving and stop talking momentarily? __Yes __No

If you stopped, how did that feel?

_____

_____

_____

What happened after you started moving again? In what way, if any, was it different than what would have happened if you hadn't stopped?

_____

_____

_____

Comment: The intention of the above exercises is to help you become more aware of your reactions and to make you more mindful of the benefits of applying the brakes, slowing down, and stopping from time to time rather than doing what comes naturally, that is, automatically.

Developing a healthy support network. We live in a society that doesn't prepare us well to live healthy lives. The same influences that have shaped us have also shaped many people we know. The people you interact with regularly will tend to influence you, so it makes sense to try to gather as many healthy people as you can into your inner circle.

Peers. Most of our peers—friends from school, friends from work, people we meet here and there—may strike us as quite normal. But how many of them are healthy, truly healthy? How many have mental and physical health as a central goal in their lives?

As we discussed above, "normal" just means what most people are, and in our society normal often includes being unhealthy. This has a lot to do with what our society teaches us about how to be successful. So beware of fitting in too comfortably with the way others are trying to live their lives. You will need to carve out your own path and create your own support network by resisting the influence of others who may have unhealthy goals or tendencies and increasing the time you spend with those who are more like-minded.

Close relationships. If you have a close relationship with a husband or wife, girlfriend or boyfriend, brother or sister, father or mother, is your relationship supportive of your goal to create a healthy lifestyle? If the answer is, "I'm not sure," have you spoken about your goal with them and asked for their support? If not, consider doing so.

To have our best chance at health, our closest relationships must be healthy. If you have concerns about your close relationships, and, in particular, if you feel you are in a relationship that may be strongly influencing you to be unhealthy, please consider seeing a counselor. Deny yourself nothing that can help you free yourself of unhealthy influences.

Summary. We have many automatic patterns of thought, emotion, and behavior that are the result of impulses, conditioning, and habits. Automatic behaviors may be responsible for how we live most of the minutes, hours, days, and years of our lifetime. Many of us develop a lifestyle around these automatic, unconscious patterns. But where such an unconscious lifestyle may lead is unpredictable.

Ultimate Recovery begins with a *conscious* decision to create a new program that will help you develop and sustain a mentally and physically healthy lifestyle. But that's just the beginning. This chapter was an attempt to help you become aware of the many automatic patterns of behavior we all have, so you can, in time, replace some of them with conscious, healthy choices about whatever confronts you in the moment. By (a) interrupting old habits again and again, (b) replacing them with healthy, intentional behaviors, and (c) creating a powerful support network, you will create a lifestyle that leads predictably to your best mental and physical health. Let's move on!

CHAPTER 7

THE MOTHER OF RECOVERY: ROUTINE

Question: "What makes the difference between those who succeed and those who fail in the community?"

Answer: "A healthy routine."

Some people think routine is boring. But how well would you be if you didn't sleep, eat, or wash routinely? Not very well at all. This is why we call routine the mother of recovery.

Routine ensures important things get done. What are the important things? (1) The things I *have* to do because they have to get done (2) the things I *love* to do because they are what make my life worth living, and (3) the *7 Recovery Practices*—whether I like them or not—because they work to maintain my mental and physical health.

Remember that a routine is not a routine until you've made the adjustments in it that you can live with and are sticking to with some consistency. Notice I said *some* consistency. No one is 100 percent consistent, and that's not necessary. What is necessary is you have developed a tolerance for some routine in your life and have a basic one you can and do follow.

Other than that, the practice of routine is having planned out then knowing your ideal routine, so you are able to return to it whenever you find you have lost consistency and your mental and/or physical health is beginning to suffer as a result.

Ease into an intentional routine. Routine is an easy concept to understand, but it can be challenging for most people to get it going and keep it going. Despite the fact that (hopefully) you have accepted how important it is, it requires discipline to maintain a consistent routine, week in and week out.

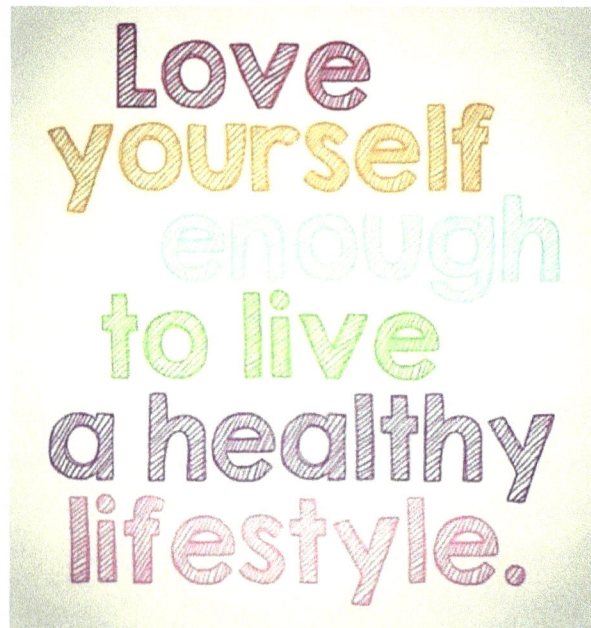
Love yourself enough to live a healthy lifestyle.

But let's be realistic. You're not a machine; you're a person. You'll never be perfectly consistent, and you don't need to be. Ultimate Recovery is about knowing how to create a healthy routine, then bringing yourself back to it whenever you realize you're off track, usually by realizing you don't feel well, are lacking in energy, are reverting to old bad habits, or you simply feel miserable. Making the connection between how you feel and how solid your routine is, is a powerful practice all by itself. Let me say that again:

Making the connection between how you feel and how solid your routine is, is a powerful practice all by itself.

Having a routine means you are doing what you've decided *needs* to be done on a schedule, you are doing what you *love* to do on a schedule, and you are routinely engaging in the *7 Recovery Practices* that promote mental and physical health. Unless you are doing these things and sticking to a schedule, you don't really have a routine.

But be patient, be gentle, and be kind to yourself. Easy does it. It's a work in progress. And remember: You can't fail if you don't quit!

It may help you to ease into an intentional routine by starting simply.

Begin by establishing a firm bedtime. Yes. Really. Mom was right! It will be difficult to get your day started at a consistent time if you aren't going to bed at a consistent time. Give this some thought. Be realistic and pick a bedtime you're likely to stick to. Don't worry; you can adjust it later. But remember that it's not yet a routine if you're constantly changing it.

CHAPTER 8

MANAGING THE ESSENTIALS: THE HAVE-TOS

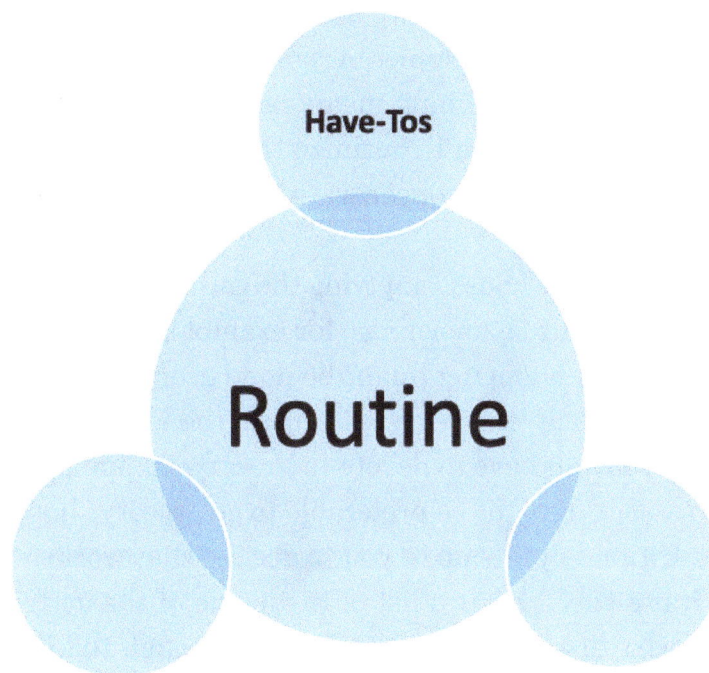

Have-Tos

Routine

Review. Ultimate Recovery begins with understanding that Life is unpredictable, uncontrollable, ever-changing. The fact that you had an injury is one example of this. But there are countless instances of unwanted changes that occur in everyone's lives, changes we are powerless to do anything to prevent. And although we can't control many of the circumstances of our life, we often can control *how we live with those circumstances*.

How a person lives is what we call lifestyle. An Ultimate Recovery lifestyle is a particular way of life, the result of an intention to be mentally and physically healthy and therefore to live according to a routine that includes and organizes three main life activities: things we *have* to do, things we *love* to do, and the *7 Recovery Practices*. In addition to providing a pathway to recovery from brain injury, we've also noted that the Ultimate Recovery lifestyle is among the surest ways to recover from any future setback Life may have in store for us.

The Ultimate Recovery lifestyle will very likely be new and quite different than any way you have lived before. It will therefore require a high level of awareness or consciousness so you can consistently choose to practice the new, healthy patterns of living rather than giving in to old, unconscious habits.

Let's look at the first category of activities in your new lifestyle.

The have-tos. This category includes activities like sleeping, bathing, dressing, preparing food, eating, paying bills, doing the laundry, shopping, cleaning, and organizing (you know that closet that is packed with stuff you never use, the stuff that is always in your way?), etc. Most of us are pretty clear on the have-tos. But failing to do one or more of these things a few times can cause problems that create stress and, if uncorrected, can become overwhelming. Establishing a routine that includes these have-tos prevents this from happening.

Some activities should occur more often than others. Sleeping and eating, for example, should be part of our daily routine. Note that having a routine means to do something on a regular schedule. Using sleeping and eating as examples, a routine would mean going to sleep and getting up at about the same time each day. It would mean eating a consistent number of meals a day at about the same time of day. If you don't routinize these have-to activities, the consequences could be fatigue, irritability, inability to concentrate, fluctuating blood sugars, spikes in blood pressure, and general chaos.

Activities like straightening up the house, emptying the garbage, and exercising can be done a few times a week. Once a week on Saturday mornings, for example, you might sit down to go through your bills and pay them. Grocery shopping might be done every other week, on a Wednesday or Sunday afternoon, rather than daily or weekly. Of course, the longer you wait between shopping trips, the more of your day you will have to devote to grocery shopping, and the more you'll have more to carry. For these reasons it might be preferable to go grocery shopping every week or even a couple of times a week. Ultimately, it's up to you to decide what works for you.

More examples of have-tos. This is a list of just some of the activities you might need to do on a routine basis in order to keep your life organized enough to have time for other things. (They are listed in no particular order.)

Eat

Sleep

Bathe

Dress

Work

Grocery-shop

Group meetings (AA, NA, etc.)

Doctor visits and therapies

Vacuum, dust, pick up around the house

Call or email family members, just to keep in touch

Call or visit close friends or family members

Wash the dishes
Cut the grass
Walk the dog
Get a haircut
Pay the bills
Take a break!

What did I leave out? Add anything below that you feel are have-tos in your life.

_____

_____

_____

Start today. As soon as you can, do the following.

1. Get a notebook. Get one that is big enough for you to write in and read comfortably but small enough to carry with you everywhere.

2. Create columns and rows for each day of the week, like this:

My Weekly Plan

Sunday	Monday	Tuesday	Wednesday	Thursday	Friday	Saturday

3. Put your wake-up time in the first row of each day and your bedtime in the last row.

4. Plug in the most important have-tos into the schedule in the order you think makes the most sense for you. (Other than your wake-up time and bedtime, it's not important what time you do the rest of the things.) Don't overload your schedule. We'll be adding other activities as we get into the Recovery Practices. For now, enter no more than three have-tos (not counting waking up and sleeping) for the same day.

5. Each morning, put that day's date on a fresh page. Copy the have-tos for that day only from your completed Weekly Plan. This activity of re-writing today's schedule can be one of the have-tos you write on your daily schedule.

6. Throughout the day, return to your schedule and cross off each item as you do it.

When does a schedule of activities become a routine? A schedule becomes a true routine only when you are sticking to it reliably without making constant changes. It takes time and effort to create a routine and self-discipline to keep it going. But do your best to stay with it. You'll know how much a routine can improve your life only after you practice it a few months.

If you find yourself wondering what's wrong with you because you're having trouble sticking to a routine, reassure yourself. *Nothing is wrong with you.* It's hard at first, that's all. Just keep doing your best to stay on your schedule day by day, week by week. Remember: You can never fail if you never quit!

Following your wake-up time and bedtime is key, and it's where you should try to achieve a high degree of consistency first. So whenever you fail to get to bed at your designated time, just try again the next day until you are usually getting to sleep at about the same time each night; the same goes for getting up at about the same time each morning.

Tip: If you're having trouble, try setting a bedtime alarm to remind you to start getting ready for bed, a half-hour before the bedtime you chose, for example.

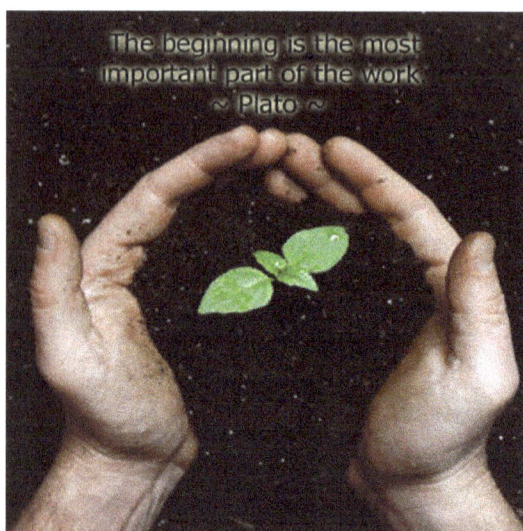

The beginning is the most important part of the work
~ Plato ~

CHAPTER 9

JOY AND SATISFACTION: THE LOVE-TOS

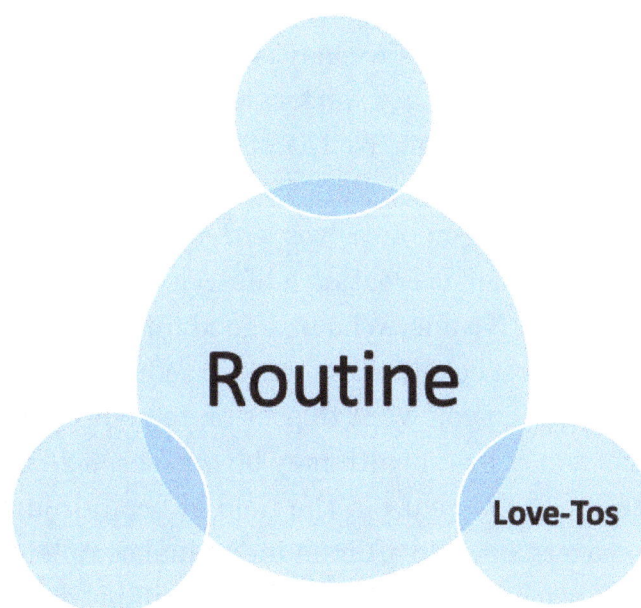

Routine

Love-Tos

You deserve to be healthy, to have fun, to have friends.

Review. Ultimate Recovery begins with understanding that Life is unpredictable, uncontrollable, and ever-changing. Your injury is one example of this, but there are many examples in everyone's life if we stop to think about them. And although it's true that we can't control the circumstances of our life, we often can control how we live with those circumstances.

How you live is what we call lifestyle. Maintaining a healthy lifestyle is the way we right the boat after being capsized by one of Life's unpredictable waves; it is a remedy for Life's ills, an antidote for the various poisons Life may bring.

A healthy lifestyle, best mental and physical health, aka Ultimate Recovery, is the result of living with the intention to maintain a routine organized around three main life activities:

things we *have* to do, things we *love* to do, and the *7 Recovery Practices*. Each of these practices is an integral part of the formula, and each one supports and strengthens the others. There is no perfecting any of them; there is only practice. I like to say, "Practice *is* perfection," because you can't fail if you never quit practicing.

Let's look at the second category of activities in your new lifestyle.

The Love-Tos. What do you love doing just for you? Answering this question needs to be taken seriously if you intend to be healthy both mentally and physically.

Coming up with activities to include in this second category of your weekly routine begins by answering the question, "What do I love doing that is also healthy for me? What gives me enjoyment, fulfillment, and a sense of pride? What really matters to me?" Determining the answers can be surprisingly challenging for a lot of us.

We tend to confuse things we love with diversion—the things we do for rest and relaxation. Let's be clear: We're not talking about watching TV, playing videogames, or hanging out. There's nothing wrong with any of these activities or others we may do for diversion—in moderate amounts. But we're talking *love* here. Most Americans are work-oriented. When we're not working, we often go into a default mode of seeking diversion. We're not as good when it comes to having "serious fun" like hobbies and avocations.

We may also confuse spending time on ourselves with selfishness. *It's anything but.* What we are talking about throughout this book is creating a lifestyle for best mental and physical health. If we succeed, who is that bad for? No one. Who is it good for? Everyone.

How we are rubs off on others, especially those we love. What do you want that to be for those who mean the most to you? What do you want to pass on to your children?

Devoting ourselves to the goal of best health may be *the least selfish thing you can do.*

An unfortunate pattern. In my years in the field of brain injury rehabilitation, I've too often seen an unfortunate pattern develop after an individual completes their rehabilitation and returns to their community. They begin to fail because they simply don't have enough to do. They may have counted on getting a job but couldn't find one. Or they couldn't or didn't want to work and had nothing they enjoyed doing to pass the time—no activity that brought them into regular contact with other people, nothing that created enjoyment and a sense of fulfillment.

Having little to do, especially if coupled with isolation, often leads to the person feeling depressed. Feeling depressed leads to other things that make matters worse. Can you guess what types of things I'm talking about? Having nothing to do can be a path to becoming angry at the world, feeling more depressed, abusing alcohol and drugs, and even engaging in criminal activity.

This chapter is about getting busy finding some healthy fun and creating a network of healthy friends who enjoy similar pastimes. This takes a little planning.

What do you *love* doing? Personal interests and meeting people are often connected, because having something you're interested in is the best way to meet people you have something in common with and making friends. It is also a critical element in staying mentally healthy by avoiding isolation and the depression that often follows.

Most of us know what we're supposed to do, because we've been told by parents, teachers, and others. But thinking of something you really love or want to do may be curiously difficult for some of us. I envy people who always seem to have something interesting to do and seem able to think of new things easily. For the record, I am not one of those people.

If this subject is a little scary for you, as it is for me, keep in mind you don't have to decide what you will love to do for the rest of your life. All you really need is to get started thinking about it. If you can come up with a few things you are willing to try, that's all that is called for at this point in your recovery.

Let me say that again: *You don't need to figure out what you love or want to do for the rest of your life, only what you're willing to try right now.*

Jennifer's method. One young woman I had the privilege to work with after her brain injury came up with the following approach for herself. Others have tried it and found that it helped. It begins by completing the chart on the next page. Take your time with it, fill it in a little a day over the course of several days. Then review it with someone who knows you well and see if they can help you add to the list.

Tip: Really throw yourself into the following exercise.

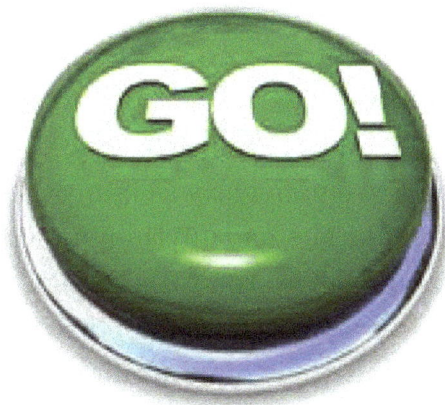

Jennifer's Method
Step 1: Identifying Dislikes, Likes, Strengths, and Things That Matter

Instructions:

- Don't put the same thing on more than one list.

- Avoid writing things that are true for almost everybody. For example, "I dislike pain" or "I like music." Instead, list things that set you apart from others. For example, "I dislike crowds," "I dislike traffic," "I like science fiction," or "I like forests."

- Think deeply about what really matters to you (column 4). For this list, think about what you think about a lot or something you have seen in your life that bothers you that might indicate something you feel passionate about.

What I **dislike a lot**	What I **like a lot**	What **I'm** *really* **good at**	What *really* **matters to me**

Having trouble? Another young woman who was in my therapy group said she just couldn't complete this chart. She didn't feel like she had anything to write. She explained that she could fill in things just to fill in things, but they weren't real to her.

This chart is challenging for most people to complete. It requires digging deeply into your past experiences and into your feelings, and many of us aren't practiced in thinking about ourselves, especially in this way. We might trivialize what we think and feel and discard many possibilities without writing them down, because we are judging our responses negatively or as insignificant. Many of us are not practiced in viewing ourselves in a positive light.

Keep at it. Dig deeper. Complete the chart. Involve someone who knows you well. Or involve more than one person. Write down your dislikes without judging them. As soon as a response comes to mind, write it down.

When you get to the last two columns, you may encounter the most difficulty. But this is where the exercise can be most beneficial. Most of us have spent a lot of our life being self-critical, so being asked to think of ourselves in terms of our strengths is unfamiliar territory.

I urge you to enter that territory. I promise you your strengths exist. Not putting the time into recognizing them is turning a blind eye to an important part of yourself. If completing the chart takes you hours or days or weeks, it is time very, very well spent.

You are worth it. Take the time to complete Step 1 before going on to the next step.

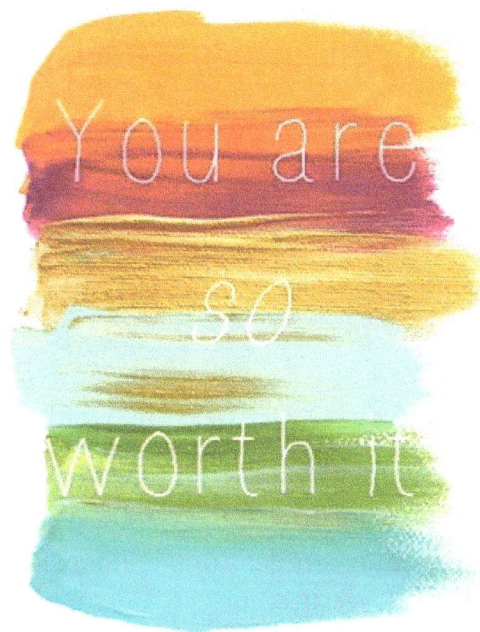

Step 2: Identifying Patterns in Your Responses

You'll need a partner for this one. Once you have the chart finished—and remember, no cheating; complete all four columns and all eight rows—look at your responses with at least three individuals whose judgment you trust who will serve as your advisers.

Ask them to look at what you have written and suggest activities you could try that (a) seem *compatible with what you wrote* on these lists, (b) that you could do *right now* (nothing that requires you to go to school for four years before you can start, for example), (c) that are *affordable and available,* and (d) that preferably *involve others.* Be as specific as possible about where a particular activity could take place (e.g., is there an organization in your community that sponsors such an activity?). Write the ideas in the box below.

> *List any activities that are compatible with your lists following the guidelines above.*
> *• That you can start preparing to do immediately. • That are affordable and readily accessible where you live. • That involve other people. Make sure to specify where this activity could take place, e.g., what organization sponsors such an activity?*

Still need help? If you belong to or attend a support or therapy group, consider bringing your completed Step 1 chart and asking the group to look at your chart to share the patterns they see in your responses. Ask for their suggestions concerning activities for you to consider. Please complete Step 2 before going on to Step 3.

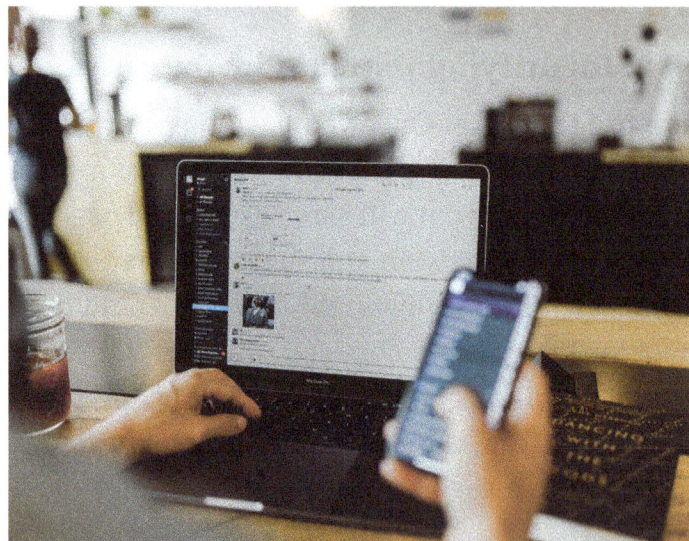

Step 3: Action

Make a call today or as soon as you can. After you've got a few activities listed in Step 2, what next step could you take to check out the activities? Who could you call, text, or email about them? Do any of the organizations have a website with a way to contact them?

See if you can make contact with at least two of the organizations associated with the activities and ask if you can arrange to go visit the locations. The most important thing is taking some action right away.

If you're stuck, who could help you think of a next step to move you toward an activity or activities? Don't go on to the next section until you have made some calls, sent some texts or emails, and made some appointments. It's important to start to find some love-tos you can try as soon as possible to develop some momentum in your lifestyle management plan. Add at least one "love-to" to your weekly schedule as soon as you have one.

THE 7 RECOVERY PRACTICES

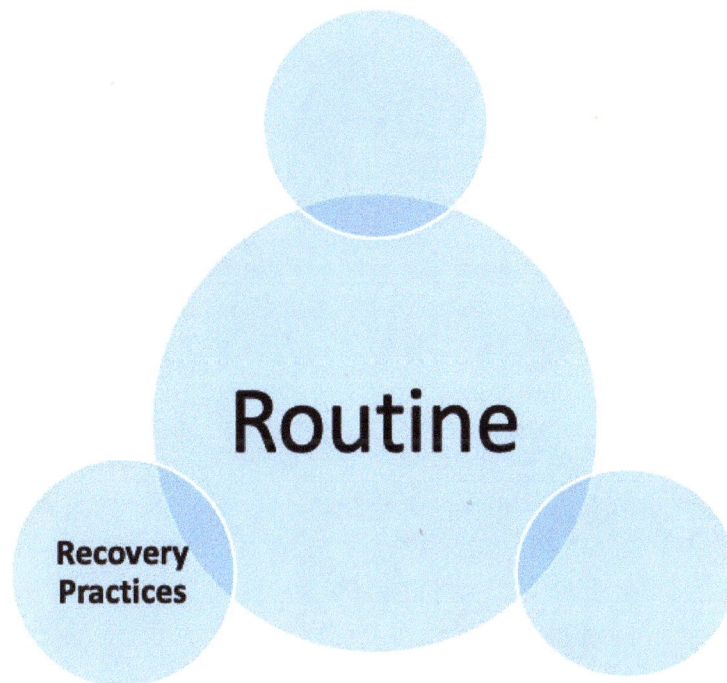

Routine

Recovery
Practices

CHAPTER 10

INTRODUCTION TO THE RECOVERY PRACTICES

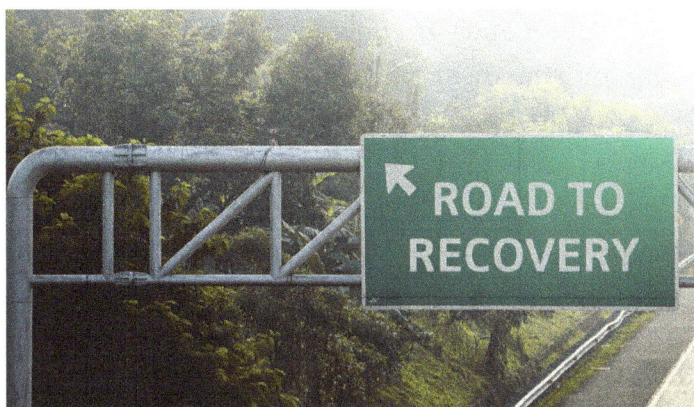

Ultimate Recovery means the creation of a lifestyle that promotes best mental and physical health.

Review. Ultimate Recovery begins with understanding that Life is unpredictable, uncontrollable, and ever-changing. Your injury is one example of this, but there are many examples in everyone's life if we stop to think about them. And although it's true that we can't control the circumstances of our life, we can often control how we live with those circumstances.

How you live is what we call lifestyle. Maintaining a healthy lifestyle is the way we right the boat after being capsized by one of Life's unpredictable waves; it is a remedy for Life's ills, an antidote for the various poisons that Life may bring.

A healthy lifestyle, best mental and physical health, aka Ultimate Recovery, is the result of living with the intention to maintain a routine organized around three main life activities: things we *have* to do, things we *love* to do, and the *7 Recovery Practices*. Each of these practices is an integral part of the formula, and each one supports and strengthens the others. There is no perfecting any of them; there is only practice. I like to say, "Practice *is* perfection," because you can't fail if you never quit practicing.

Let's look at the third, and final category of activities in your new lifestyle, the Recovery Practices.

1. **The Practice of Fitness.** The Earl of Derby is credited with having said, "Those who do not find time to exercise will have to find time for illness." It is well-accepted that regular exercise promotes brain recovery. And regular resistance and aerobic training will make you feel great. Combine exercise with good sleep and a reasonable diet and you'll be ready to take on the world!

   There are six more practices that focus specifically on mental health.

2. **The Practice of Realism.** By this time in your life, you have no doubt been filled with ideas about what your life is or should be. Some of these ideas are valuable, some less so. A few common ones are downright destructive. If you have unrealistic expectations, you can only be disappointed. If you have realistic expectations, you will be able to keep a firm grip on what is practical, attainable, and healthy, and as a result, create a more satisfying life.

3. **The Practice of Self-Acceptance.** If you don't think much of someone, will you exert yourself on their behalf? What if you don't think much of yourself? It isn't likely you will do what it takes to achieve Ultimate Recovery if you really don't accept and care about yourself. In a future chapter we will discuss just how surprisingly common shame and self-loathing are. The Practice of Self-Acceptance will help you move past these and other emotions that can get in the way of Ultimate Recovery.

4. **The Practice of Gratitude.** It is much more natural for our brains to focus us on what's wrong in our lives rather than on what's right with them. Therefore, we need to practice seeing what is good and what is working in our lives, or we may come to believe our lives are failing in some fundamental way despite how obvious our successes are to everyone else.

5. **The Practice of Clarity.** Our everyday modern world can be chaotic and confusing. We are assaulted with sights and sounds and experiences of all kinds, all day, every day. Within us exists another world of thoughts and emotions that can be even more chaotic and make us even more confused. Journaling, the Practice of Clarity, is a simple but powerful way of sorting through the chaos and achieving tremendous clarity.

6. **The Practice of Serenity.** What would you give for some serenity? Well, all it really takes is practice. The Practice of Serenity is meditation, not for religious purposes but for health and healing. Meditation has been shown to promote the

natural healing of the brain, to improve attention and memory, and even increase brain mass.

7. **The Practice of Presence.** Your life only ever occurs here and now. Yet it is surprisingly easy to neglect what is here and now—including ourselves and the people in our lives—due to all of the distractions inside and outside us that stimulate us and disrupt our connection with the present, causing us to focus on the past and the future.

    Not surprisingly, this leads to feeling disconnected. The simple practice of mindfulness can make a huge difference in your emotional outlook and keep you focused on the only time your life actually exists, in the present.

When you begin to incorporate these practices into your daily routine, you will be doing the best you can to do the best you can. What more is there? This is why we say:

You can't fail... if you don't quit!

CHAPTER 11

SLEEP, DIET, AND EXERCISE: THE PRACTICE OF FITNESS

For our purpose, fitness will refer to three activities: sleep, diet, and exercise. Let's take them one at a time.

SLEEP: Getting what you need. Let's talk about sleep first. Here's what Samuel Johnson, the great 18th-century English writer, had to say on this topic:

"Sleep is a state in which a great part of every life is passed. ... And once in four and twenty hours, the gay and the gloomy, the witty and the dull, the clamorous and the silent, the busy and the idle, are all overpowered by the gentle tyrant, and all lie down in the equality of sleep."

—From *The Idler*, by Samuel Johnson, 1758

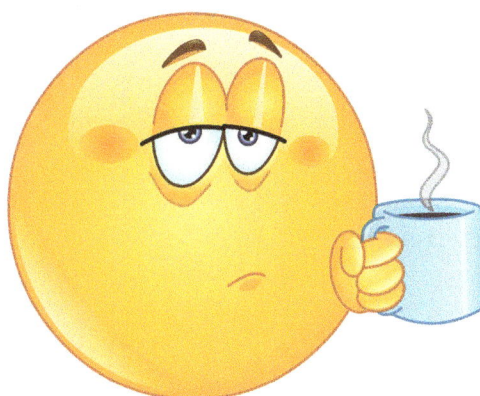

"All lie down in the equality of sleep." Here are some facts about sleep that may surprise you:

- Millions of Americans have occasional sleep problems.

- About one in six have chronic insomnia and consider it a serious problem.
- Some neuroscientists have claimed that up to 100 percent of survivors of traumatic brain injury may experience some degree of sleep disturbance.

Insomnia refers to habitual sleeplessness. We'll use the term "sleep disturbance" to include folks who have occasional sleep problems in our discussion. There are four forms of sleep disturbance:

1. Difficulties falling asleep

2. Difficulties staying asleep

3. Poor-quality sleep

4. A combination of any or all of these.

Sleep can affect everything in your life. When you haven't gotten enough sleep, nothing works right. Energy, mood, attention, reasoning, problem-solving, learning, memory, work performance, and relationships might all suffer. The good news is that these all might also improve when sleep improves. So be honest with yourself when evaluating whether you are having problems in any of these areas that could be affected by poor sleep patterns. To be sure, you may want to ask someone who knows you whether they notice that you yawn or seem inattentive during the day, whether you seem unable to focus and complete tasks, and/or whether you have a short fuse and are easily irritated.

Conditions that we have had for a long time are likely to escape our notice. We develop blind spots leading to denial then to chronic impairments that lead to lifelong problems.

Common Causes of Sleep Disturbance

- Unrealistic sleep expectations, like believing you have to get 8 hours every night
- Inappropriate scheduling of sleep
- Trying too hard to sleep
- Consuming too much caffeine or drinking it too close to bedtime
- Inadequate exercise or exercise too close to bedtime
- Breathing problems
- Stress and anxiety
- Drug or alcohol use
- Depression
- Pain

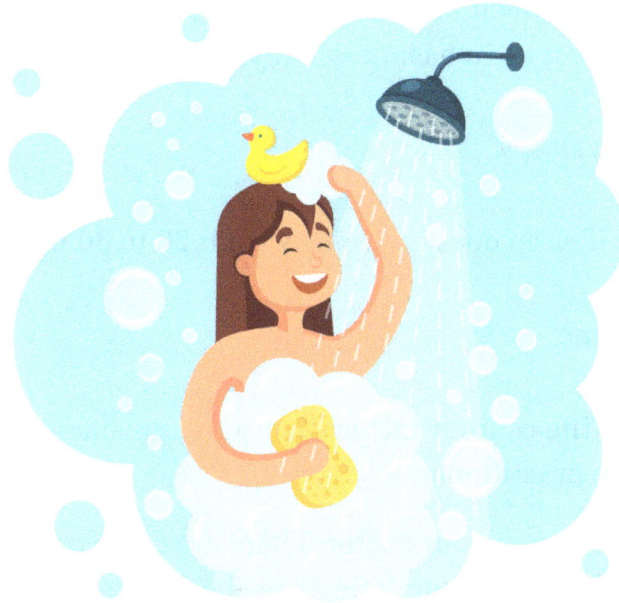

Sleep Hygiene Tips

1. Keep regular bedtime and wake-up hours, even on the weekend.

2. No caffeine-containing foods or drinks 3 hours prior to bedtime.

3. No heavy exercise 3 hours prior to bedtime.

4. No alcohol, nicotine, or heavy meals within 2 hours of bedtime.

5. Avoid bright light exposure near bedtime.

6. Avoid exposure to light from TV, computer screens, e-readers, or smartphones before bedtime.

7. Stop TV viewing of disturbing or stimulating TV shows at least 1 hour before bedtime.

8. Foster a quiet, pleasant sleep environment—a cool room and soft lighting.

9. Have a relaxing bedtime routine—taking a warm shower, thinking about things you're proud of or happy about (think hard—there are some), doing meditation or yoga.

10. Use the bed for sleep—which means no watching TV, working, or reading. If you watch TV in your room, sit in a chair when you watch.

11. Go to bed only when sleepy.

12. Go to another area if sleep does not come within 20 to 30 minutes.

13. Avoid daytime napping.

14. Don't take any over-the-counter medications or supplements unless approved by your doctor or nurse practitioner.

Still having problems? Talk to your doctor. There are other causes of sleep disturbance that require medical attention. Consider completing the checklist on the next page and taking it to your next doctor's appointment.

Sleep Self-Assessment Checklist
For Discussion with My Doctor

Name _____   **Date** _____

After each statement, circle True or False.

Sleep onset. I have difficulty falling asleep. It takes 30 minutes or more for me to fall asleep.

True   False

Sleep maintenance. I have difficulty staying asleep. I believe most nights after I have fallen asleep, I wake up for more than 30 minutes.

True   False

I wake up in the early morning before I want to get up, and I can't get back to sleep.

True   False

Poor-quality sleep. I don't feel rested after sleep.

True   False

Effects of sleep. I experience:

Daytime fatigue	True	False
Impaired performance	True	False
Mood disturbance	True	False

Reminder: This checklist is to share with your doctor or licensed healthcare practitioner.

HEALTHY EATING

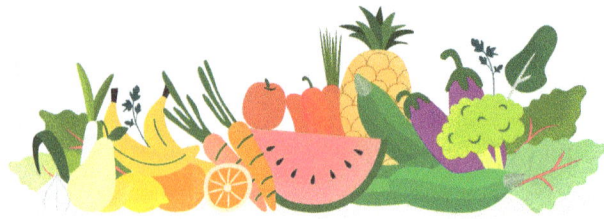

DIET: Everything in moderation. There are some basics that most people ignore or forget about what we eat. As with so many of the healthy living principles and practices, a little change in your diet could go a long way to helping you reach your Ultimate Recovery goal(s).

A vicious cycle. Few countries have more information available concerning dieting; at the same time, few countries have more diseases associated with poor nutritional habits. Our eating habits are often locked into a chain or cycle of habits that reinforce each other. Changing one tends to change others—but trying to change any of them tends to be resisted by the others.

Let me give an example. Suppose you're eating because you're bored or depressed. It's common to turn to food in times of stress. Before you know it, you start to develop the habit of inactivity that goes along with eating. Then you give up the exercise or level of physical activity you were used to. Soon you find that your circle of friends and people you have daily contact with have gotten smaller. Over time you feel isolated, negative, and lonely.

So you eat some more. You turn to comfort foods, such as those with high sugar or fat content. You put on weight. And you increase the motionless activities that now consume hours each day, while you're eating more and more and feeling worse and worse. Less and less activity, less and less social contact lead to more and more isolation and depression.

Humans are full of these vicious cycles. Being mindful and intentional about our life and going after something worthwhile in a patient, self-affirming manner is the way to break a vicious cycle.

Take some time to really consider the following guidelines about healthy diets. Which of them can you start putting into place *right now?*

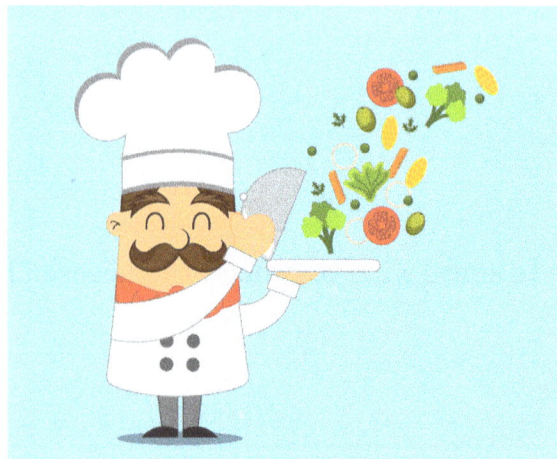

Guidelines for Eating Yourself Well. These simple suggestions will work for most people to get them started on a healthier eating regimen. As with everything in this book, if your doctor's advice is different than what is recommended here, follow your doctor's advice.

1. **Eat a variety of foods**—Don't let your favorites become the only thing you eat. Add something you don't usually eat a few times a week. Think about cheese, milk, yogurt, pudding, different fruits, vegetables, cereals, nuts, breads, rice, seeds, noodles, and meats.

2. **Maintain a healthy weight**—If you're trying to lose, lose a little at a time. Avoid going to extremes. Exercise a little more. Don't skip meals. Eat a little less. Cut back on the most fattening foods a bit. Don't eat or drink near bedtime. Whatever you do gradually is more likely to become part of a lasting lifestyle.

3. **Choose a diet low in fat, saturated fat, and cholesterol**—If you have a habit of eating lots of chips, cookies, ice cream, fries and other fried foods, doughnuts, butter, etc.—cut back.

4. **Choose a diet with plenty of vegetables, fruits, and grains**—Cut back on meat. When you see a vegetable or fruit in the café or supermarket, buy some. If it's on your plate, take a bite. If you're dining out and they're available, think about ordering more vegetables and skipping the fries.

5. **Reduce your sugar**—Enough said. And remember that sugar hides in lots of foods you may not realize, so read the labels.

6. **Reduce your salt intake**—If you're adding salt until you can see it, you'll become beef jerky. Salt is bad, bad, bad. And it hides everywhere, so read the labels.

7. **Reduce your caffeine intake**—If you have a seizure disorder or take psychotropic medications, this is important. Caffeine can reduce the effect of these medications. Like sugar and salt, caffeine hides in lots of drinks, so again, read the labels.

8. **Eliminate alcohol**—If you have had a problem in the past with alcohol, if you have a seizure disorder, or you take psychotropic medications, this is essential.

EXERCISE: Get Moving. Physical exercise means exertion, raising your heart rate, perspiring a bit. But before you do anything that raises your heart rate or makes you perspire, make sure you have your doctor's blessing.

Going to a gym and working with a trainer is great if this is possible. But there are so many other ways to increase the amount of exercise you get each day and to get some exercise routinely— things you could easily build into your routine today. With a little thought, I'm positive you can think of some. List a few below that may work for you given your resources. Remember to think big but start small.

_____

_____

_____

_____

_____

_____

_____

Include whatever form of exercise you prefer into your routine.

Remember:

Those who have no time to be healthy will need to find time for *illness*.

Think big but make small changes, a little at a time.

Small changes will lead to Ultimate Recovery!

CHAPTER 12

KEEPING IT REAL: THE PRACTICE OF REALISM

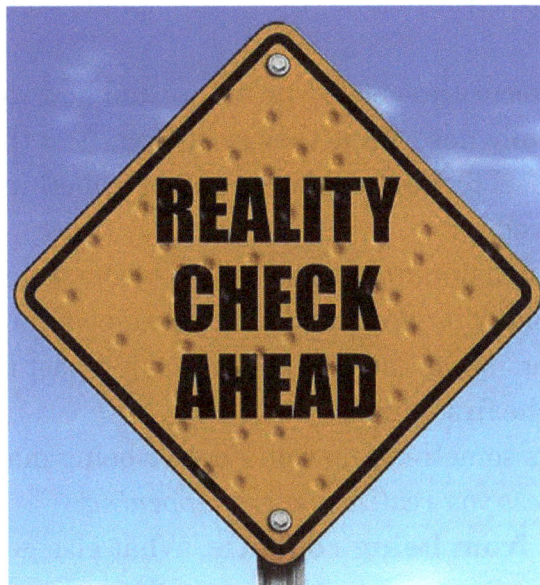

What is "realism?" Realism is defined as:

"The attitude or practice of accepting a situation as it is and being prepared to deal with it accordingly."

Realism doesn't come naturally. We have heard and perhaps have said to others, "You have to be realistic!" Why do we need someone to tell us this? Why is it difficult to keep it real? Part of the problem is that being realistic doesn't come naturally. Our minds are creative power tools able to imagine just about anything. Add to this the automatic function of our thinking, and our imaginations can easily run away with us. When this happens, we can begin to prefer what exists in our imaginations to reality.

I'm not saying imagination is the problem. Imagination is great. Our capacity for imagination has served us well by permitting us to solve difficult problems, create art, and design buildings and spaceships, to name just a few accomplishments of the human mind. But in our everyday life, this same powerful ability can confuse us and sow dissatisfaction with our life as it is. I said our minds are creative power tools. All we need to do is to learn to use that tool to our best advantage.

As with everything, it's a question of balance. A little dissatisfaction with how things are can stimulate our creativity and motivate healthy change. But taken to an extreme, dissatisfaction with our life may become so pervasive that we lack any peace of mind. Obviously, that's not a prescription for best mental and physical health!

Marketing and imagination. One of the main reasons we can become chronically dissatisfied has to do with the effect on our imaginations by modern marketing. Capitalizing on the ease with which we can become engaged in fantasy, marketers fill our heads with ideas about how their products will make us better and happier. They do their best to *create* dissatisfaction with what we have and convince us that what they're selling is the remedy.

"Wouldn't you be happier with our swanky brand X sports car? Wouldn't you be a better cook with our super-duper, multiprogrammable, internet-capable electric cooking pot? Don't you *deserve* the best?"

Marketers often prey on insecurities about who we are and how we measure up to others. They try to convince us that we really need what they're selling. And their messages can be hard to resist. We can easily be led to feel like we're missing out on something essential for our happiness if we don't buy this or that product.

As a result of our powerful imaginations, superheated by marketers, we can easily come to feel that our life as it is, is perpetually *inadequate*. We find ourselves on a treadmill of desire always running after "new and better" so we can feel better and get past the feelings of dissatisfaction that marketers put there in the first place.

And because there's always something new and better being made and marketed, there's no getting off that treadmill *unless you realize what's happening.*

Beliefs that prevent us from being realistic. What else gets in the way of choosing to be realistic and live in reality? One common barrier is that many of us are full of ideas we got growing up about the way Life is *supposed* to be, *could* be, and *would* be if we were only smart enough, tough enough, talented enough, rich enough, lucky enough, or worked hard enough.

Many of us have come to believe that we can and should bend Life to our will. But this isn't realistic. We are limited beings. Life is bigger than any of us. Sure, we should do our best to reasonably improve our life. But when we try to bend Life to our will, and we inevitably fail, we may think there is something wrong with us. Or worse, we may come to believe there is something wrong with Life itself. Then the real suffering begins.

Most of all, realism means avoiding extremes of thought. Avoiding extremes lets us keep solid ground beneath our feet. Let's examine some popular myths. Each one is an example of extremist thinking that can lead to having unrealistic, unhealthy expectations for our life.

The "I can do anything I put my mind to" myth. No, you can't do anything you put your mind to. Neither can I. I need air to breathe. Without it, I will die. I need to eat. Otherwise, I will die. I cannot survive beyond a certain range of temperature. Otherwise, I will die. There are so many conditions on which my life depends that I can do nothing about, no matter how much I put my mind to it. The same is true for you.

To believe you can do anything you put your mind to is an unrealistic, unhealthy fantasy. No matter how much I put my mind to it, I cannot leap tall buildings in a single bound, bend steel in my bare hands, or change the course of mighty rivers. Superman can do such things, but he is a comic book character not a real person.

No matter how much you put your mind to it, there are many, many more things you cannot change than the things you can. If you believe you should be able to do anything you put your mind to, and you don't get the results you expected, you may come to believe you're powerless, which is another myth we'll cover later. You may feel guilty or ashamed that you haven't been able to master Life. Are you ready to give up this comic book version of life?

Being realistic means we must accept the possibility of failure. Being realistic means we know we will never change the big realities of Life: We will get old (if we're lucky). We will get sick. We will die. Everyone does. These are the most basic realities of human existence. These realities are only depressing if we have made a habit of denying them, as many of us have.

Being realistic means accepting that to be human is to be limited by many, many things. This does not mean we cannot succeed at making the most of our talents and achieving some of the goals that matter to us. It just means that we must consider our limitations and abilities carefully, so we choose our goals wisely. It means we have to plan carefully, so we make the best use of our opportunities and resources.

The "my life should be exceptional" myth. This is a continuation of the above belief. The unrealistic belief that you are or should be all-powerful might cause you to have unrealistic beliefs about Life itself, including that you can and should be able to create an exceptional life.

It's not likely you're exceptional. It's not likely you are *exceptionally* smart, *exceptionally* talented, *exceptionally* rich, *exceptionally* lucky, *exceptionally* fast, or *exceptionally* anything. How can I say that? Because if most or even many of us were exceptional, "exceptional" wouldn't be exceptional—it would be normal, it would be average, it would be ordinary!

If most of us were exceptional, "exceptional" wouldn't be exceptional— it would be ordinary!

And what's wrong with ordinary anyway? How did "average" become a dirty word? How did "normal" become insufficient. It isn't. They're not. But many of us have been told that to be normal, ordinary, or average isn't good enough. And we believed it. Maybe you still do.

Ordinary just means to be like most people. Average is what most people are. Normal means the same thing. Normal, average, ordinary, usual, common, typical—all mean pretty much the same thing. What's so bad about being any of these things? Nothing, unless you were brought up to believe these are not good enough.

The real lives of real people are mostly normal, average, and ordinary. From time-to-time Life can be dramatically wonderful or dramatically painful. We may have times of great joy and other times of great suffering. Life—everyone's life—can include all of these things and more. But for most of us, our life occurs in the in-between places, between the extremes of wonderful and terrible, of agony and ecstasy, of light and heavy, of magical and dismal, of triumph and tragedy.

We may not even notice how true this is, because we are so busy noticing the dramatic times. The times Life is great. Or the times Life is miserable. Even when we're not living through such times, we tend to be thinking about them. And this is how we miss out. This is how our normal, average, ordinary, basically good lives pass us by without us having noticed, without our having truly lived.

Being realistic means coming to terms with the normality, averageness, and ordinariness of our life. It means not resenting, resisting, or regretting these qualities. In fact, it means seeing that a normal, average, ordinary life is something we can all be grateful for. The gift of Life itself.

The "I am powerless" myth. This is the opposite extreme of the kind of thinking we just covered, and it's every bit as unrealistic. Although you never have and never will have total control over your life, it's not true that you have *no* control. For example, it may have been true that you had no control right after your accident, when you were in the emergency room, and perhaps for the weeks or months after that when your life was dependent on medical attention. But where are you now? Aren't you somewhere between the two extremes of "no control" and "total control?"

Aren't you closer to normal, average, and ordinary than when you were first injured? That's called progress. That's the goal. That's where real life happens.

We can plan and problem-solve and carry out our plans and solutions. We can make meaningful changes in the quality and direction of our life. You picked up this book to make a change. Keep reading and use what you learn, and you will indeed experience the result of your real personal power.

The "pain is bad" myth. Pain is a part of Life. And by "pain" I mean any kind of discomfort, physical pain, delay, inconvenience, dissatisfaction, disappointment, or emotional upset. These are all part of real life. But we tend to react to these common, normal, average, ordinary occurrences with shock, disbelief, resistance, anger, and sometimes rage, depression, or hopelessness just because we believe they shouldn't be happening.

When we have such reactions, we move ourselves beyond pain to suffering and misery. By suffering and misery, I mean *what we do to ourselves in response to the pains* that are part of real life. What if we could simply remain in reality and in touch with whatever pain we are experiencing in a particular moment? What if we could remain calm and resist the extreme reactions I mentioned above?

Is it possible that by doing so our painful experience might be transformed into something more tame, more tolerable? Would a day in which we remained calm, present, and in touch with our moment-to-moment experiences (the good and the bad ones), just letting them happen without any big reaction, be a better day?

One last myth: "Practice makes perfect." Doesn't it? Doesn't a little or a lot more effort make the difference between failure and success? Sometimes. As long as your objective is realistic in the first place and you have a well-thought-out plan for achieving it.

But practice doesn't really make perfect. That's because perfect doesn't exist. It is only an idea. No matter what you or anyone else comes up with that is supposedly perfect, someone else can come up with something better. So perfect is nothing more than someone's idea, and it is always subject to an upgrade by someone else.

Practice makes perfect is yet another saying that suggests we have control over our destinies. But this kind of control is an illusion. Change is the only thing you and I can count on. The very fact of your injury is proof of your limited control over things. There are countless other such proofs all around us. Change, sometimes dramatic change, is just a fact of everyone's life.

No amount of effort will allow you to surpass the limits we've talked about. No amount of effort will likely allow you to make your life exceptional. Those few individuals among us who possess exceptional talents and who do manage to accomplish exceptional things, even they must learn to accept the fact that most of their lives occur in the normal, average, ordinary range. If they can't accept that, they suffer. The ranks of the rich and famous are full of examples that attest to this truth. All of us, ultimately, will grow older, become sick, and die, despite anything we accomplish.

The Practice of Realism challenges us to recall and to keep recalling that we are impermanent beings living in an impermanent, ever-changing world among other impermanent beings. What if we could develop the habit of returning to this realization again and again? What if we could not only accept impermanence but embrace our vulnerability? Wouldn't it lead us to recognize our kinship with all the things and people in our life and to appreciate them more?

Practice _is_ perfect. Ultimate Recovery is based on the principle that practice is perfect. This means that as long as you continue to practice, you will continue to improve. You will continue to become healthier, mentally and physically. But don't take my word for it. Find out. Take the plunge.

You have nothing to lose but needless suffering.

Change, the ultimate reality. Virginia Satir, the noted social worker, psychotherapist, and author, famously stated, "People prefer the certainty of misery to the misery of uncertainty." This is another way of stating how primal is our need to have stability in our life.

But change is constant. Many of the things we want are things we think will create a happy stability in our life. There's nothing wrong with working to make improvements in your life, as long as you don't fall for the fantasy that stability can be achieved, that change can be resisted, and that loss can be avoided.

"Change is the only constant in life."

—Heraclitus

The affirmation on the following page is one I encourage you to make part of your daily routine. It contains the principles of the Practice of Realism and several other Practices contained in the pages to follow. Reciting an affirmation regularly is a way to take deeply to heart what we have been studying and to make it a part of your daily life.

Affirmation on
REALISM and SELF-COMPASSION

My Life is a Life at sea. The sea will have its way. I know I cannot control it. My Life must tilt this way and that because the sea has waves. So, like a sailor, I must develop my sea legs and learn how to give in a little to the waves, to go with them, and then to recover my balance, again and again.

I embrace this rocky Life at sea because the rocking means Life.
Only a sinking boat doesn't rock.

So I am a sea creature too, a part of it, part of Life happening. All of it—*all of us*—moving and changing together: the wind, sea, clouds, seabirds, fish, insects, microbes, people. No winners and no losers, just the rocking, the change. Just Life.

My past does not govern my future any more than the wake of a ship governs its course. Life is Now. Only, always, ever, Now. Whatever is done is done with. Whatever is yet to be, may never be. Nothing is certain but Now. It is what I do Now that matters. Though I cannot control Life, I can control my response.
I am Response-Able.

I practice mindful connection with each experience, each precious moment. Each sacred Now. I practice deep, compassionate connection with others and with myself. Those who behave badly need the most compassion, the most help.

When the person behaving badly is me, I too deserve compassion—never impatience, condemnation, or self-punishment. I practice self-acceptance, not shame, over how I am or what I am. I accept myself with all my talents and triumphs, all my shortcomings and failures, even while I seek positive change. With all that I love about myself and all I may regret, I am perfect—perfectly alive, *perfectly human*. Both failures and successes are just rocking.

The least selfish, most Response-Able thing I can do is to be clear about what I need most to be healthy and satisfied today then to work toward it, if only a little bit every day. The better I care for myself, the more worthy I will feel; the more worthy I feel, the better I will care for myself.

With every little success, I enrich myself.

When I enrich myself, I enrich everyone around me. Taking care of myself and others in this way is the essential highest good, not because it will make me rich or famous, but because we need each other, and our survival depends on it.

I will not fall into the trap of suffering needlessly by insisting bad things should never happen. At least not for long.

I will not allow my emotions to run wild when I get knocked down by one of those waves. At least not for long. I will not lash out, numb out, withdraw, or escape with drugs, alcohol, or other distractions. At least not for long. I will try first to slow down and stop. I will try then to remain present with what is, with what I feel, and with Life as it is in the moment, rather than with what I wish it would be. I will try to remember to breathe and remember that this too—whatever "this" is that troubles me—will pass.

I will try neither to hold back my emotions nor give them power over me. I breathe and relax with whatever I feel, positive and negative. I let my feelings, my Life, flow in and through me.

And I vow to develop my balance, to live with the greatest appreciation for this magnificent ship, the wondrous sea, wind, fish, seabirds, insects, microbes, and people, the brilliant sun, and the entire universe that peers through the night sky and rocks right along with the rest of us!

This is my Wisdom. This is my Life. In this I am whole. In this I am satisfied.

Summary of the Practice of Realism.

- If we believe that we are or should be in control of our life, we are on a direct course to needless suffering and misery.

- If we believe that pleasure should last or pain can be avoided, we are on a direct course to needless suffering and misery.

- If we believe that being normal, average, or ordinary is insufficient, we are on a direct course to needless suffering and misery.

- If we believe that to be normal, average, or ordinary is to have failed in some way or that having a normal, average, ordinary existence means *Life has failed us,* we are on a direct course to needless suffering and misery.

- If we believe we have no control over anything, we are probably already suffering and miserable—needlessly.

- Consider reciting the Affirmation on Realism and Self-Compassion as part of your daily routine.

Suffering and misery are fairly easy to generate because most of us have been programmed to believe one or several of these unhealthy, unrealistic ideas that lead directly to them. But it's possible to change and begin to reverse these beliefs and achieve a more balanced, more realistic point of view and experience greater health and joy as a result. This is the objective of the Practice of Realism.

Simply put, being realistic is to become acquainted with Life as it is. It means making a choice to reject constantly running after more and better. It means making a choice to accept and embrace a mostly normal, average, ordinary life. If you can make these choices, you will have taken a giant step on the path to best mental and physical health—Ultimate Recovery.

If and when you decide to make the choice to live realistically, you may be surprised at how good that life—your life—can be.

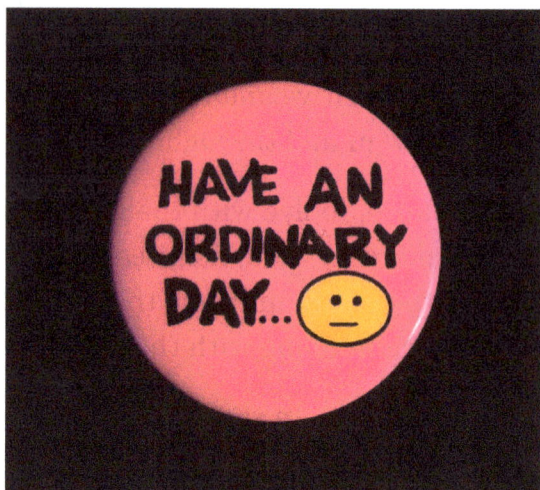

Reminder: I must periodically restate that if you disagree with anything I have to say here or elsewhere in this book, if your life is just fine the way it is, or if you are generally content and satisfied with your life, put down this book and carry on!

Chances are, if you felt that way, you wouldn't have picked up this book and read this far. So let's continue.

CHAPTER 13

BECOMING YOUR OWN BEST FRIEND: THE PRACTICE OF SELF-ACCEPTANCE

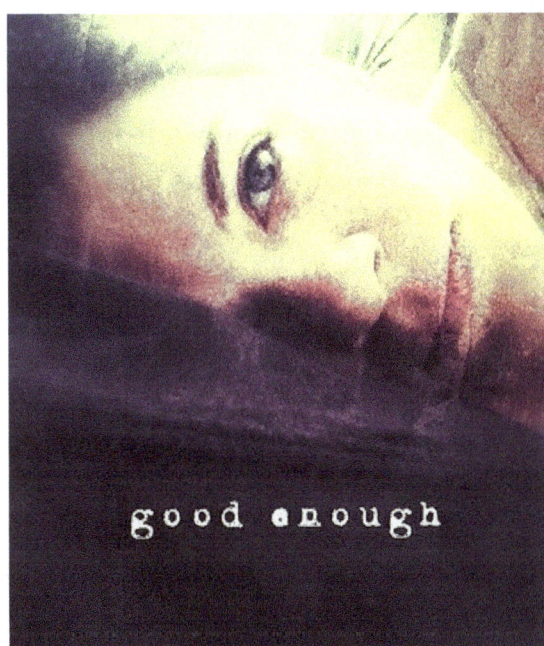

"I'd rather be whole than good."
—Carl G. Jung

The Practice of Self-Acceptance. The simple truth is that most, if not all, of us have things about ourselves we don't like, aren't proud of, or are frankly ashamed of. That is part of what it means to be human. We can always imagine a better us, but the difference between what we are and the person we imagine we can be may cause us to feel dissatisfaction, guilt, or outright shame. There are lots of reasons why we get involved in this kind of imagining, but the point is, there are a lot of us who dislike aspects of who we are and wish they were different, more, or better.

Once again, if you can relate to this, you are not alone. This common trait makes it challenging to ever accept ourselves. Yet accepting ourselves is a basic prerequisite for our mental and physical health.

Carl Jung's statement—"I'd rather be whole than good"—is worth thinking about. Interestingly, the words "wholeness" and "health" come from the same root. To be whole is to be healthy; to be healthy is to be whole. And to be truly whole means accepting the good, the bad, and the ugly: the parts that feel complete and sound as well as the parts that feel tattered and wobbly, the parts that perform beautifully and those that may not function at all. Can you imagine ever being capable of that level of self-acceptance? Keep reading!

I have never met a person without self-doubt. I have heard the most amazing people—people who are accomplished writers, athletes, doctors, clergy members, chefs, therapists, scientists, artists, and effective parents—say they have lived most of their lives with a sense of "not being good enough." Some believe that the very reason they accomplished what they did was due to their self-doubt. Because of it *they felt compelled to prove themselves.*

So self-doubt may have gotten a bad rap. Doubt can open our mind to different perspectives that can enable and motivate positive change and growth. But what struck me most is that these same highly accomplished folks said that no matter how much they accomplished, the feeling of not measuring up, of not being good enough, of not being able to fully accept who they are, even of feeling frankly ashamed of themselves, never really left them.

I think that's the real shame, and it's one of the reasons I wrote this book.

What may be wrong with you is that you think there's something wrong with you.

Acceptance. Do you accept that you're reading right now? I didn't ask if you accept *what* you are reading but whether you accept *that* you are reading. Do you accept that you're alive? Do you accept that to keep reading you'll have to turn the page or scroll down? So let's be clear: Acceptance has nothing to do with liking or disliking or with agreeing or disagreeing. Acceptance simply means to recognize the truth or the reality of something, someone, or some situation. Self-acceptance means to recognize the truth, the reality about ourselves.

To be whole is to be healthy. To be healthy is to be whole. Self-acceptance as a health practice means recognizing the truth about *all* of you—the things you like and the things you may not. Here's some good news: Accepting the truth about yourself may not be as scary as you think. The truth may surprise you and be easier to acknowledge than you imagine.

Some common obstacles to self-acceptance. It may help to examine some of the reasons many of us have such a hard time accepting our whole selves. Some are quite common. Here are a few:

- **Fear**—fear of seeing or letting others see our shortcomings. Most such fears are unfounded.

- **Empty praise**—If we were praised for every little thing we did as a child, we may experience resentment, anger, and painful self-doubt when we experience adult life, which is devoid of such continuous praise.

- **The media**—We are constantly barraged by images in the media of people who are presented as normal, everyday people. But models used in advertising are mostly selected because they are abnormally good-looking, impeccably groomed and dressed, and always appearing happy and in command; they are pictured in luxurious surroundings in a crowd of adoring friends. Consciously or unconsciously, we may adopt these idealized images as normal and the standards against which to evaluate ourselves. If you feel you must measure up to what you see in the media, self-acceptance will be out of reach.

- **Perfectionism**—We have discussed the saying "practice makes perfect." Perfection is just an idea, and it has no existence outside the mind. We can always imagine a better idea, which is why attaining perfection is never possible. So if you must have perfection in order to accept yourself, self-acceptance may be impossible.

- **Self-shaming**—Conscience is an inner voice that guides our actions toward what we believe is right and good and away from what we believe is wrong or bad. It is this capacity that causes us to want to do the right thing. This is a positive and healthy motivation when it causes us to do our best to live up to standards of ethical behavior. Doing your best to live up to your standards is great. But we go too far when we shame ourselves for failing to always live up to them.

  When we shame ourselves, we can become chronically depressed or angry and impair our ability to grow, do better, and be healthy. Ideals serve a purpose if they motivate us to act better. They can become destructive when we fail to take credit for our efforts. This may happen when we become rigid and perfectionistic, when ideals become absolutes that must be obeyed at all times.

Deeper sources of self-doubt, guilt, and shame.

- **Guilt over having been injured**—It's not uncommon for victims of brain injuries to feel responsible for having had their car accident, for having fallen, even for having had a stroke. People blame themselves, believing that if they had only done this or that, they could have avoided their fate. Perhaps there is some truth to it. But the whole truth is that we have much less power over our life than we like to imagine. Self-acceptance will remain out of reach as long as you believe having been injured was your fault and you deserved it.

You didn't deserve to be hurt. No one does.
You deserve to be better. Everyone does.

- **Unresolved grief**—This form of self-denial is another major barrier to accepting ourselves. When we shut ourselves off from the feelings that accompany a significant loss, we shut ourselves off from a part of ourselves.

    Loss is the most human and most humanizing of all experiences. Having lost does not make you a loser. Loss is what we all have in common. Who do you know who hasn't experienced it?

    Healthy grieving should eventually lead us to being able to feel, letting hurt in, and accepting our vulnerability and our need for others as well as our strength and resilience.

    Review Chapter 3 if unresolved grief is an issue for you. Engaging the Practice of Self-Acceptance may require seeking professional help. If you think you may benefit from professional help from a psychotherapist, why not explore it?

- **Addiction**—Persons who suffer from addiction often report feeling inadequate and unworthy. Addiction may be a cause of feeling inadequate, it may be the result of feeling this way, or both may be true. Once a person begins to depend on drugs or alcohol to feel OK, he or she may feel more and more guilt and shame for the damage they inflict on themselves and others. This pattern cannot be broken until the person becomes clean and sober and is able to think clearly, feel honestly, and learn to live in a sober, healthy way. If you're committed to your sobriety, you have taken a giant step toward engaging the Practice of Self-Acceptance.

- **Unresolved trauma from abusive relationships**—If we grew up in a home where one or both parents were alcoholic, abusive, or neglectful, or if we witnessed abuse of a sibling or parent, if we had to live through our parents' angry divorce, or if we have been in an abusive adult relationship, it is not uncommon to feel somehow responsible for what happened to us—even though in reality, we were the victim. Once again, the Practice of Self-Acceptance may require professional help. Please don't hesitate to seek it out.

- **The curse of the neocortex**—I'm going to end this section with my favorite. The neocortex is the learning, thinking, problem-solving area of the brain. It is the part of our brain that allows us to imagine. It is the part responsible for landing on the moon, all the wonders of medicine, the *Mona Lisa,* and everything else you'll find in a museum. Wonderful, right? Well, of course. But it is this very brain that also allows us to imagine a better self. That too is good, as long as we can manage to like who we are all the while we're imagining a better model. But we may experience unwarranted shame if we allow imagining who we could be to make us feel bad about who we are. This is what I refer to as the "curse of the neocortex."

Recovery is not the way to self-acceptance.
Self-acceptance is the way to recovery.

Self-loathing and our inner critic. Every one of the above obstacles to self-acceptance typically results in the creation of a harsh and vocal inner critic. Have you ever heard him or her putting you down? If not, you may need to listen closer. Most of us have one. And it's this inner critic that does the real damage to our capacity to accept ourselves. As long as our inner critic is allowed to operate, we are practicing self-abuse and moving steadily away from self-acceptance and Ultimate Recovery.

I have a friend who is very sensitive about his weight. He told me about some cruel treatment he received from peers when he was an adolescent, all because he was. My friend is now an adult, no longer overweight, and accomplished in his career field. Yet he remains highly sensitive about his weight. Of course, one of the reasons is how much pain he suffered as a child, even though that was a long time ago.

My friend has also confided that every time he gets out of the shower, he sees himself in the mirror and thinks, "Ugh. I look terrible. I need to lose some weight." Every time he puts on a pair of pants that are a little snug, he admits his first thought is, "Man, I'm fat!" Just seeing another man looking fit and trim gives him a twinge of jealousy followed by a disparaging thought or comment about himself. Do you see what's happening?

My friend has been repeating that old criticism that began in childhood. He has been repeating the abuse he suffered long ago, keeping the wound open, not allowing it to heal by *practicing* self-loathing. Because he's been practicing it for so long, I suspect he's quite good at it. I suspect his criticisms come easily and can be particularly harsh.

As a result, he has become what he has practiced all these years—disrespectful, of himself.

So what does he do to turn things around? "Go to the gym," you might say. But if his motivation for going to the gym is that he disrespects himself as he is, he's in for a battle. Part of him will arrive at the gym determined to tone up and trim down. But his self-disrespect will show up in many forms and erode his motivation to continue. Self-loathing is a great motivation—for quitting.

As long as we are self-loathing, our inner bully will be at war
with the healthier side of us that wants us to be well.

Self-disrespect and self-abuse aren't skin deep; they're much deeper. He may manage to lose some weight and look better to others, but it's doubtful he'll really like himself enough to maintain his gains. If he slips for a few days, misses the gym, or puts on a few pounds, that inner bully will let him have it and grind him down. In the face of such abuse, such self-abuse, he may well conclude it's not worth the effort to get in shape, and he'll give up.

Recovery is not the path to self-acceptance. Self-acceptance is the path to recovery. Practice self-acceptance to recover because you believe you deserve it and because you believe in your power to help others by first helping yourself.

Exercise: Identifying Your Inner Critic. Self-loathing and the self-abuse that results from it need to be confronted and changed. For that to happen, we have to first become aware of these negative practices. For the next 24 hours pay close attention to what you're thinking and feeling as you go through your day. This exercise asks you to detect instances of self-abuse and record at least one of them.

Instructions. Pay close attention to feelings in your body during the next 24 hours. Any time you feel ill, tense, achy, in pain, fatigued, or nervous, it might be an indication you have been quietly practicing self-criticism. When we negatively evaluate ourselves, there may be some constriction or some tightening in our gut or elsewhere. Learn to tune in to what you're feeling and ask yourself whether it is associated with some form of self-criticism. Record your experience in the spaces below.

What did you feel in your body and where did you feel it?

_____

_____

Where were you when you recognized your demeaning self-evaluation?

_____

_____

What was happening at the time that might have triggered it?

_____

_____

What were your specific self-critical thoughts?

_____

_____

Reflect on your relationship with yourself. We all have a relationship with our self. We are all two points of view. I am two "me's. You are two you's. I am the me who thinks, feels, speaks, and does, and I am also the me who judges my thinking, feeling, speaking, and doing. I am both the judge and the subject of my judgment. This applies to you as well.

What is your relationship with yourself? Are you aware of conflict between you and you? Are you at odds with yourself? Do you pick on you? Call you names? Make fun of you? Taunt or tease you? Harshly judge yourself? Is there a fight going on inside of you?

Take a few minutes now to write down your thoughts about these questions: What is your relationship with you? Are you more like your own best friend or more like your worst enemy?

What do you practice that caused you to answer the way you did?

How do you pick on yourself?

Let's see if we can make a change. What is good about you? This may be tough at first. But fill the space below. Don't go on until you have.

Listening to yourself through journaling and mirror talk. What would it feel like if someone told you, "I don't care what you feel. Keep it to yourself." It wouldn't feel good. It would make you feel uncared for, cut off, alone, and perhaps angry. And this is exactly what we do to ourselves when we deny our feelings and fail to show enough interest in them to fully listen to what we are feeling.

The practice of denying our feelings and failing to show enough interest in them to say or write them are practices of self-*dis*respect. If we don't have loving, caring interactions with ourselves, we will certainly have self-critical ones. Our relationship with ourselves will be predominantly self-critical because we become what we practice. As always, the choice is yours.

Listening is magic. When we really listen to someone, including our self, it is an expression of concern, acceptance, and caring. It is a rare and precious thing to be really listened to, especially by our own self.

Some of us may lack the emotional vocabulary to understand what we "hear" when we try to get in touch with what we feel. Here are some emotion words for you to review to see if any of them help you with the listening exercises that follow.

Anger	Surprise	Disappointment	Vulnerable	Hate	Envy	Dread	Content
Happy	Excitement	Frustration	Satisfaction	Grumpy	Irritation	Anxiety	Pride
Fear	Disgust	Abandonment	Gloomy	Helpless	Horror	Cheerful	Relief
Sadness	Thrill	Betrayal	Lonely	Love	Panic	Delight	Shame

Listening to ourselves helps us feel cared about by the one closest to us—the person in the mirror. There are two ways to practice listening to yourself.

- **Journaling**—writing about how you feel—is one of the most powerful ways we can practice listening to ourselves. To be able to think of something to write on the blank page, we must first become quiet and "listen" to the feelings and ideas that circulate within us. (We'll also talk about journaling in some detail in a later chapter.)

- **Mirror talk**—looking yourself in the eyes in a mirror and asking, "How are you? What are you feeling just now?"—is another way of listening to ourselves. This may strike you as odd, but don't knock it until you've tried it! Mirror talk allows you the opportunity to listen directly to yourself through speaking and to feel the feelings that come along with the words, thus becoming intimate with the person looking back at you.

Exercise: Listening to Self Through Mirror Talk. Keep in mind that this mirror talk exercise is an exercise in self-respect. Do it in private, so you don't have to feel self-conscious. You may be surprised to discover that even alone it requires some courage to do this exercise. But it will be worth it to do it. You'll need a mirror, notebook, and pen.

There are four parts to this exercise.

Part 1: Once you're alone, stand or sit still in front of a mirror. Look directly into your own eyes. Hold your gaze as steady as you can; this is important.

Ask yourself the following question, out loud, maintaining eye contact with yourself as you do. Ask the question as if you are really concerned and want an answer:

"What do you feel most deeply, right here, right now?"

Re-ask the question if you need to until you have an answer.

Part 2: Once you have an answer, say it to yourself, out loud, while continuing to look yourself in the eye.

Part 3: Now look directly into your own eyes and say:

"I care about *you*.

I *care* how you feel.

I am here for you."

Part 4: Once you have done all of the above, write about how this exercise felt as you were doing it. Write as much or as little as you wish to. Use extra paper if necessary or write in your journal if you have one.

There's actually one more important part.

Part 5: Repeat daily. Add this exercise to your weekly schedule.

Summary of the Practice of Self-Acceptance.

- First, catch and redirect your negative self-talk.

- Second, keep adding to your "what is good about you" list.

- Third, and most important, talk to the person in the mirror regularly—as if you were her or his own best friend.

- Consider reciting the Affirmation on Realism and Self-Compassion (in the last chapter) as a part of your daily routine.

By now you may be clear about your intention to recover and to create a lifestyle devoted to your best mental and physical health. This chapter has been about making space to nurture deep caring for yourself to help you keep going.

When we allow ourselves to feel for ourselves, we are expressing interest in our own journey and interest in taking care of ourselves, come what may. Allowing ourselves to feel our deepest feelings is an act of commitment and love for the person who looks back in the mirror.

Note: If you are suffering the aftereffects of child or adult emotional trauma, be willing to find and receive the help you need and deserve. Make an appointment with a psychotherapist. If you don't know one, ask your doctor or other healthcare professional.

CHAPTER 14

EMBRACING YOUR LIFE: THE PRACTICE OF GRATITUDE

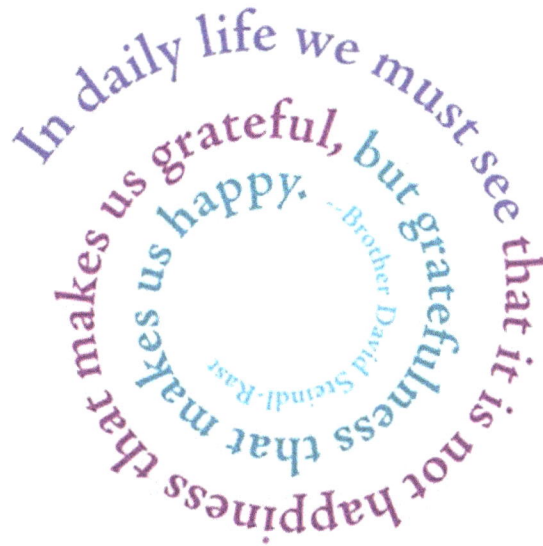

In daily life we must see that it is not happiness that makes us grateful, but gratefulness that makes us happy. —Brother David Steindl-Rast

The negativity program. The science of evolution tells us that many of our physical, emotional, and mental traits developed to provide us with a survival advantage. For example, opposable thumbs, color and depth perception, the fight or flight reflex, and our brain functions all helped us survive and thrive as a species. Even the emotion of fear, while disconcerting, is an evolutionary creation that makes us cautious and helps us avoid dangerous situations.

We tend to notice what's wrong, what's broken, and what we want but don't have more readily than we notice what works well, what's good, and what we have in abundance. And this tendency toward seeing the negative may be associated with evolution as well. It may give us a survival advantage to see the negatives in that it may help us keep our cupboards stocked and our houses clean and steer us away from calamities like forest fires and famine. So negative thinking may be quite useful in some ways.

But there's no doubt that this negative thinking can make us feel bad about ourselves or our lives. Like so many things, it's a question of balance.

Survival Requirements vs. Health Requirements. The following chart illustrates the natural traits that evolution has built into us to ensure the survival of our species and the traits that don't come naturally, the ones we have to create if we want to achieve our best mental and physical health.

Survival Requires	Mental & Physical Health Requires
Noticing what's broken and fixing it.	Noticing what's working and being grateful for it.
Noticing what's missing and providing for it.	Noticing what you have and being grateful for it.
Noticing what's wrong and putting it right.	Noticing what's right and being grateful for it.
Noticing what's a threat and eliminating it.	Noticing that you're safe and being grateful for it.
Noticing what could be improved and improving it.	Noticing what is perfectly sufficient and being grateful for it.

Evolution isn't concerned whether we enjoy best mental and physical health, only that we're alive. Noticing things we can be grateful for certainly feels better than negative thinking, and feeling better is what Ultimate Recovery is all about. But if negativity really is programmed into us, what can we do about it?

This is an important question, because if we aren't grateful to be alive, why bother with recovery? Why bother with anything? Yet how can we reprogram ourselves so we can be more positive, notice some of the good stuff and not just the bad, and become more appreciative of and grateful for our life?

Please realize that we're not promoting seeing the world through rose-colored glasses. We are simply promoting a more balanced view of Life and living that is required if we are to achieve our best mental and physical health.

The answer, as we've said before, is a matter of practice. Because of our brains' basic programming, we don't need to practice negative thinking. It comes quite naturally. But if we want to enjoy the rewards of a more balanced view of our life, we'll need to practice noticing the positives as well. The way to change is simply to practice.

You become what you practice.

Noticing basic goodness. For the next 5 minutes, make a list of the things that are basically good right here, right now. Start with the easy stuff such as noticing you have a chair to sit on and that you are well-protected from the elements as you sit where you are reading this. Don't think too much—just notice what is obviously good. See how much you can come up with. Stick with it for a full 5 minutes. Look at the time now and begin.

What if you practiced noticing things that are basically good in this way at the end or the beginning of every day? Would that change anything? What do you think? How would it change things if, instead of being a slave to the basic programming of your brain and being mostly pre-occupied with wants, needs, worries, and regrets, you practiced noticing all you have, how little you really need, how abundant your life is, and how much you have accomplished?

What if you did this every day for a year? Do you think it would make a difference? Is it worth the effort to find out?

Gratitude journaling. Gratitude is the emotion of being grateful for something or someone. Gratitude has long been recognized as a characteristic of healthy people. But as we've seen, it may be much easier to be negative because we have a built-in program for it.

Negativity can become a monster that overtakes our life. It can spread like a disease through-out our mind, heart, words, and actions. Negativity is a breeding ground for criticism, anger, and depression. It can even spread to others.

The practice of gratitude, on the other hand, can be as simple as being grateful you woke up this morning, grateful the sun came out or rain fell to water the flowers, grateful the floor you walk on is level and you have indoor plumbing, grateful for having felt a cool breeze on a hot day, or grateful for having enough food to eat.

Gratitude can also become a habit. Gratitude is like penicillin for negativity. It is not the prac-tice of seeing the world through rose-colored glasses. It is the habit of noticing that never does a day go by where there is not something or someone to be grateful for—all you need to do is pay attention and be on the lookout for these things and people. They're everywhere! And gratitude also spreads—to contentment, satisfaction, and happiness.

Developing the practice of gratitude journaling is a way to reprogram yourself to pay attention to things you probably don't see most days. Try keeping a gratitude journal. Take 5 minutes at the beginning or the end of the next 2 days and write a few things you are grateful for. You should easily be able to fill the rest of the page. Use extra sheets as needed.

Reminder: Don't proceed until you have continued the exercise above for at least 2 days.

Elevators, flush toilets, a hot meal, a birthday greeting, street signs, a pair of gloves in winter. Did you include any of these kinds of things in your lists? All are the result of a lot of effort by many people over many years to make your life and mine more convenient and comfortable.

There are hundreds of examples of this kind of support we can be grateful for from others. But we rarely reflect on all the things we receive from the creativity, labor, and dedication of others. We tend to take these things for granted and focus instead on what we don't have. For reasons we've already mentioned, negativity comes naturally. Left unchecked, this kind of thinking creates an imbalance in our perspective and distorts reality.

The Practice of Gratitude is the practice of acknowledging all the support we receive. It is a practice that can restore the balance between the things we feel we lack and the beneficence of the world we inhabit. Consider the following: Imagine what would happen if you spent 5 to

10 minutes every morning and evening expressing gratitude for experiences you had that day? What effect do you think it would have if you kept that up for a year? Then imagine what would happen if you spent the same amount of time each day complaining and you kept that up for a year? Get the point? The thoughts we fill our head with will tend to create the reality we live in.

Gratitude balance sheets. Most people are familiar with balancing a checkbook. You keep track of the money you put into your account, and you deduct the money you spend. What's left is your balance—how much (or little) you have.

I'm aware of the things I do that I'm proud of and the things I do I'm not so proud of. But that still leaves a lot out. There are many things I do for others that they may appreciate but that I may not notice. The Practice of Gratitude becomes most powerful when we add to it a sense of responsibility to give back at least some of what we get from others.

To help you be aware of the difference between what you get and what you give, add to the two lists below each day for at least 3 days.

Things I Received	Things I Gave
A place to live, air to breathe, light, sidewalks, food to eat, a smile, etc.	I held a door open, gave someone directions, smiled and greeted someone, etc.

Things I Received	Things I Gave

Reflection: Your Feelings About Gratitude. Take some time to write down how you felt while making your lists. Do your best to write out the specific thoughts and feelings you had.

_____

_____

_____

_____

_____

_____

Summary of the Practice of Gratitude.

- It's more natural for our brains to notice what's broken, what's wrong, and what we don't have. In other words, it can be surprisingly normal to be dissatisfied with our life.

- Still and all, if we aren't grateful to be alive, why bother with recovery? Why bother with anything?

- Without downplaying things that may need improvement in our life, it is worth practicing being able to see what's working well, what's good, and what we have enough of. In this way we provide ourselves with a more complete picture of our actual lives and with reasons to feel more positive about them.

- In this chapter we discussed how to create a gratitude journal, a way of training our brain to see good things it's probably missing. Make journaling a part of your routine, daily, weekly, or even monthly. Decide what suits you best. It's consistency that matters.

- A powerful companion practice is at the end of the day to think of several positive things you're grateful for, things that occurred that day. If you can't think of anything at first, stick with it until you come up with something. Remember that it's natural to see the negative. But with practice, you'll get better at noticing the positives. Try doing this as soon as your head hits the pillow. Keep it up for 30 days and see how you feel. You may find that you sleep more soundly by ending your day with positive thoughts.

Healing

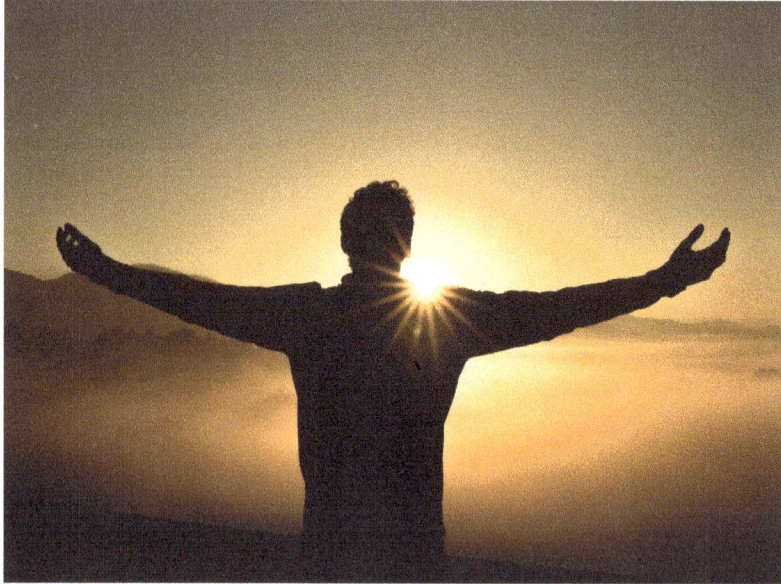

Feeling is the first step
to healing our wounds.

Sharing with someone who
cares is the second.

Accepting who we are, losses
and all, is the third.

Gratitude for what we have
is the fourth.

CHAPTER 15

JOURNALING: THE PRACTICE OF CLARITY

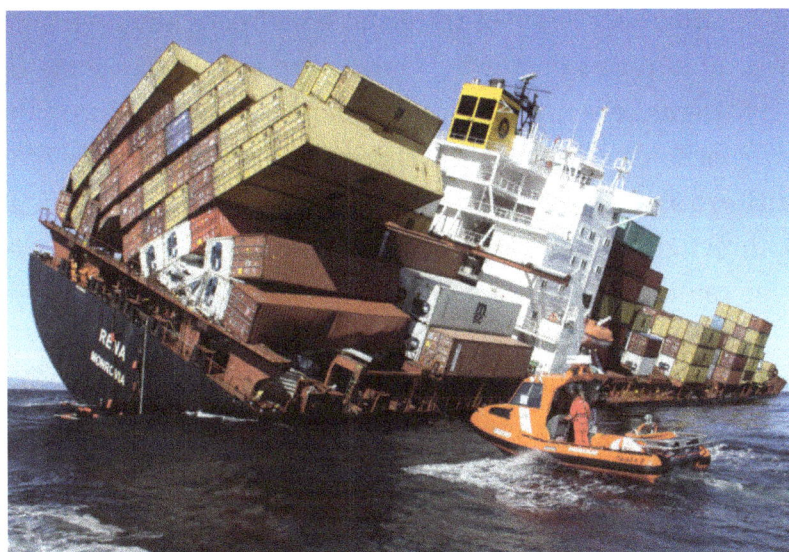

Have you ever felt better after you talked with someone about something that was bothering you? When you did this, do you recall if you also felt a little *clearer* about the experience? Perhaps clearer about what actually happened, why it happened, or about how you handled it?

Many of our thoughts tend to be thought fragments, gut reactions, and images. But once we start putting thoughts into actual words, all that changes. When we talk to someone else, we are forced to select the right words, to complete sentences, and to put it all in a logical order so the person listening can understand us. As a result, our feelings and thoughts take on a shape they probably lacked while they were floating about in our heads.

Consider this example: I go into a store and encounter a rude salesperson. During the encounter, I have a number of emotions. I don't express them though because I'm just trying to get my stuff and be on my way. But once I leave the store, strong feelings surface as a result of the disrespect I experienced and perhaps because I didn't speak up and put the person in their place. But this is all mostly a muddle of emotions as I hurry on my way—a hearty stew of outrage, anger, and embarrassment but no clear thoughts other than a few headlines like "What a nasty person!" and "I'll never go into that store again!"

When I get home, I put away my groceries, fix myself a cup of coffee, and call a friend. During the conversation I share my store experience. For the first time I'm putting it all into words. It feels good to have someone who is willing to listen to me.

As I tell all the gory details, I add some background for my friend: "It was that store that just announced they're going out of business because they're opening a bigger store over in Bigger Town. Do you know it? It has mostly minimum-wage jobs. But a lot of folks work there because they don't have a car to travel to a better-paying job. So I guess that means some of these folks will be out of work. The salesperson didn't have any right to take that out on me. But I guess she might have been on edge."

Did I have all these thoughts and all this clarity at the time of the event? No. It was only when I put my experience into a story that I could see the big picture and gain some understanding and perhaps some perspective for the rudeness I had at first taken so personally.

Conversation can do that, which is one of the great benefits of having friends to talk to. Writing can be even more powerful in terms of gaining clarity and relief after some upsetting experience. We all have the capacity to make sense of a lot of things in our life if we take the time to reflect by writing about our experiences. That's where journaling, the Practice of Clarity, comes in.

Journaling is high-quality thinking. The activity of reflective journaling requires us to engage in purposeful, directed, sustained, logical thinking. Until or unless we challenge ourselves to try it, we may never realize how powerful a practice it can be. Some people love journaling almost immediately. Others warm up to it slowly. Some never do.

Sometimes the difficulty is with the mechanical act of writing, of course. For example, if you have hand tremors, hand weakness, or incoordination, it may be difficult to write. Occupational therapy may help working through mechanical problems.

The objection some people have to journaling betrays the difficulty they have just thinking. Intentional versus automatic thinking can be difficult! But more often, resistance to journaling is due to the effort required in recalling. When someone says, "I can't think of anything to write about," they usually mean it's difficult to recall things they thought, felt, or did. But the more you journal, the better your recall may become. Journaling is recalling and thinking, recalling and thinking. You become what you practice.

Many things happen each day that offer opportunities for reflection, insight, and clarity. But until you actually make time in your routine to reflect, chances are there's a significant amount of your life slipping by unnoticed, unrecalled, and not fully experienced. On the other hand, once you begin to write about your experiences, you may be truly amazed to see how much more grounded and connected to your life, to events, to people, and even to yourself you become.

Reflection requires that you take the time to stop and stand back a bit, then put whatever you're writing about into some kind of logical, complete form. It begins with focusing your mind enough to recall something you may have been barely conscious of at the time.

Writing is the practice of *consciousness*. The more you write, the more conscious you will become. Guaranteed. But as with all advice given in this book, it's up to you to be the judge.

But be a fair judge. Write consistently, every day or two, for a week. Notice how you feel before and after you write. At the end of the week, you will be in a good position to fairly judge whether journaling deserves to become a regular practice on the road to best mental and physical health.

Recommended practice of reflective journaling. Living with clarity depends on clear thinking, and clear thinking requires practice. Start today to write at least a paragraph each morning, afternoon, or evening. You'll need a notebook. You can keep your gratitude journal in the same book. You may benefit from following the prompts below to get you started.

> Note: A prompt is a question that helps get your writing started. Use one of the following if you can't think of anything to write about.

- What am I grateful for?
- What is it I am resisting?
- How am I practicing self-acceptance?
- What do I feel right now?
- What did I receive today?
- What did I give today?
- What does "You become what you practice" mean to me?
- What does "You can't go back; you can only go forward" mean to me?
- What does "a wake-up call" mean to me? Have I had one—how so?
- What new awareness(es) have I received as a result of being injured?
- Of what value to myself is this new awareness? To others? To my community?
- "Best mental and physical health." Is this a meaningful way to think about my recovery now? Why or why not?
- What are the one, two, or three things I do on a regular basis that constitute my recovery routine?
- We are healthier in connection with others, but many of us have learned to separate ourselves from others. How do I separate myself from others? Why?
- How do I give to others?
- An example of my anger and how I dealt with it, is ...
- How does my anger serve me?
- How have I grieved?
- What do I do to keep from receiving love from others?
- How do I have to clean up my act?

- What I regret and the lesson I have learned from that experience are …
- I have approached losses in the past by …
- How I would like to approach loss now is …
- The most important thing I have lost in my life and how I have responded to it are …
- What I fear losing most now and what I do with this fear are …
- What I don't want to write about is …
- The ways I have been brave in my life are …
- The ways I am good enough are …

It's hard to know how you will respond to reflective journaling, but I strongly encourage you to give it an honest try and to add it to your recovery routine. The more you do it, the better you will get and feel and the more logical and insightful your thinking will become.

CHAPTER 16

MEDITATION: THE PRACTICE OF SERENITY

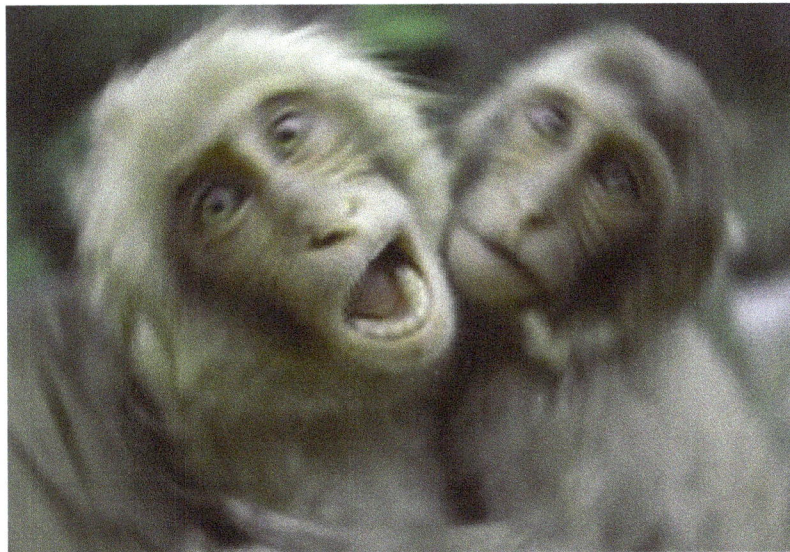

Who couldn't use a little serenity? In today's world there's so much stress. There are so many sources of stress. And one of the main sources is our very own mind.

Inside our mind are these crazy mental monkeys that jump from one idea to the next, from one emotion to the next, all day and all night. We sometimes confuse their incessant chatter with thinking. But a lot of what goes on in our heads is not actually thinking, just these brain monkeys doing what they were programmed from birth to do automatically.

Our brains are programmed to be powerful automatic-association machines. The monkeys are the brain's programming in action. If I say "big," one of your monkeys calls out, "small!" If I say "tall," another monkey shouts, "short!" If I say "up," yet another monkey yells, "down!" You don't have to actually think to come up with any of these responses. It's the monkeys or, more accurately, our brain's automatic programming.

Just about anything I say or do in your presence, just about anything you see, hear, taste, touch, or smell will cause some immediate association. Our brain monkeys are always ready for action! When harnessed, this powerful association machine can be useful for learning, problem-solving, planning, and creative thinking of all kinds. But the problem is, even when we aren't trying to learn, solve problems, plan, or create, the monkeys are still jumping about, screeching out associations and reacting to everything and everybody, including their own chatter.

So even when we manage to not react physically, our monkeys force us to react mentally and emotionally, creating stress, which over time can create chronic health problems like high blood pressure.

Unfortunately, our brains don't come with an off switch. Yet, if we're to get some peace and quiet, we must somehow get the monkeys to stop. Until we do, they carry on more or less incessantly. And we're trapped in the cage with them!

Serenity is freedom. If our mind automatically reacts to everything and everyone, we are constantly being dragged about. We are a slave to our own minds. But if we can learn to quiet the monkeys, we can get that much needed peace and quiet. With even more practice, we can open the cage door and gain our freedom from them anytime we want.

Until then, we won't have the freedom to *not* react or even to delay our reaction, which would give us time to think.

Good judgment requires time.

Bad judgment or no judgment? Let's expand on a topic we introduced earlier. Sometimes the best choice is to delay any response until we have had the opportunity to observe more carefully what is going on, accurately hear what someone is saying, understand what they want, or discern what a situation requires. Extra time can amount to a big difference. And sometimes the best reaction is no reaction.

Good judgment requires time. But we don't have the freedom to stop or delay a reaction as long as our monkeys are in charge. Without the freedom to choose how and when we will react, what we usually consider bad judgment may actually be no judgment at all. When the monkeys are in charge, we can't stop, look, listen, and think. We are forced to react again and again with little or no thought or deliberation, without exercising any real judgment at all.

Slow down. Take your time.

The magic of slowing down. While there is no off switch for the automatic activity of our brains, it is possible to slow things down so we are able to function more deliberately. That alone can create a magical difference in the way we function in the world.

In our daily life, slowing down our movements, our speech, and our breathing, even for a few seconds, can make it easier to see what is present in any particular situation, to reflect, and then choose the right next move (which may be no move at all). Can you think of a time when—had you been more in control of your monkeys—you might have said or done nothing, at least for a moment or two, to give you time to think, and you would have been better off as a result?

Try to recall one situation where not reacting would have been the best response and write it down.

_____

_____

_____

_____

_____

_____

_____

_____

_____

The importance of perspective. Try this. Pick up your cell phone or any small object and hold it close, right in front of your eyes. What do you see? Can you see anything at all? Doesn't the object block out the sight of almost everything else? Can you even see the cellphone or object?

If you can put a little mental distance between you and whatever it is you're thinking about, you can realize how actually small it is *in relation to everything else that is going on.* Isn't that what is meant by putting things in their proper perspective?

Is this a mountain or a molehill?

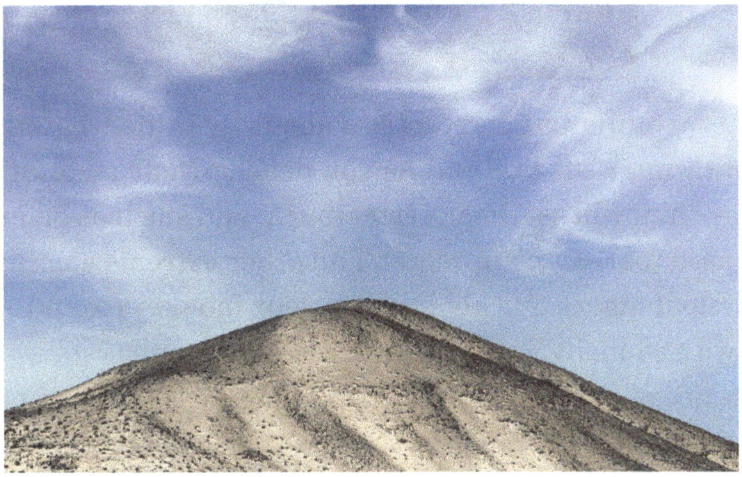

You'll have to step back to know.

A molehill can look like a mountain until you step back and create some space to see it compared with its surroundings. When we bring what we're thinking or feeling about up so close that it blocks out everything else, it can seem like a single thought or emotion is much bigger than it actually is or even that it is all there is. Isn't this how we blow things out of proportion?

When we learn to create space for ourselves simply by slowing down, we often see that whatever is bothering us is much smaller than we first thought. Stepping back allows us to realize most things just aren't that big a deal.

Taming your monkeys through meditation. Meditation—the Practice of Serenity—involves training your brain to slow down, to become still, so that taking a mental step back from whatever is going on becomes easier. Meditation is a powerful means of taming our monkeys.

Meditation can be challenging. Just sitting still might be difficult at first. We've always got a mental itch to scratch. But with repeated practice we can achieve stillness. This will help us feel calmer and able to breathe and act more consciously and wisely—and see if action is required at all. When we can calm ourselves and take that mental backward step, the problem, whatever it is, will often seem a little or a lot smaller, a little or a lot more manageable.

Or, once again, perhaps you will realize that it's not a problem at all.

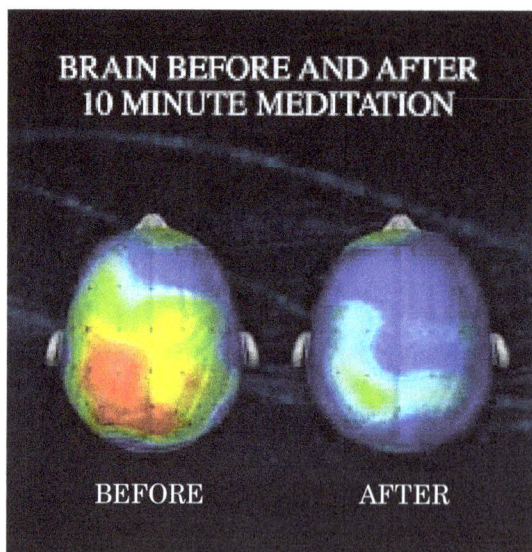

BRAIN BEFORE AND AFTER
10 MINUTE MEDITATION

BEFORE   AFTER

Most people develop very different perspectives about their life when they begin to gain even a little mental control through meditation. As you develop your meditation practice, you'll be capable of feeling calmer. You will see, hear, taste, touch, and smell as before, but you'll probably notice more than you used to. Fear, pain, regret, and other extreme emotions probably will arise less frequently and dissipate more quickly because your monkeys aren't stirring things up and cluttering your mind with so many automatic mental reactions.

Meditation, the Practice of Serenity, is the practice of quieting the mind's automatic activity, becoming still, and stepping back mentally to create space to observe clearly what is—and doing this again and again. But just how do you still your mind and take that backward step? Let's talk about puppies instead of monkeys for a minute.

Learning to sit-stay. If you're a dog owner, you know about the challenge of teaching a puppy to sit and stay. It's one of those skills that is good for both the pup and the owner. Being able to sit and stay might keep the little thing from running into the street and getting run over. And once the pup learns to sit and be calm, the owner can relax a bit.

Like the puppy, our brain needs to be trained to be still (sit) and be present (stay). It doesn't happen without practice. Meditation is the method for accomplishing this. The method itself is quite simple and has been shown to have many benefits, including reduced blood pressure, improved sleep and attention, easier-regulated emotions, and even increased brain mass.

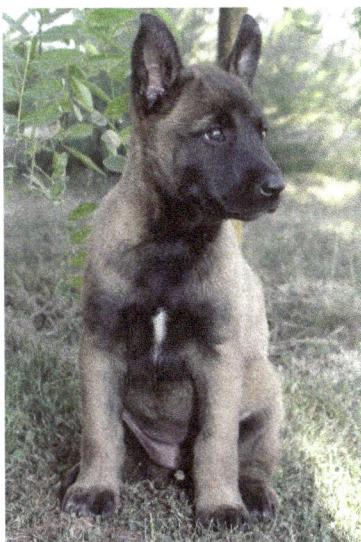

How to meditate. You'll want to prepare first.

- Decide when you will meditate.
- Decide where you will meditate—find a quiet place, free of distraction, if possible.
- Ask those you live with to give you some privacy for your meditation time. Put a "Do Not Disturb" sign on the door if necessary.
- Turn off your TV, phone, computer, and anything else that creates distraction.

Then sit and follow these guidelines:

- Sit comfortably with your hands resting loosely in your lap.
- Sit tall, meaning sit up as straight as you can, with a slight upward stretch of your spine.
- Try to anchor your mind to something you can focus on, such as counting your breaths.
- Count 1 for a complete breath cycle (an in breath and an out breath)
- Repeat this for 10 breaths, then start over.
- Sit still. Be gentle. *Slooooow* down.

- Try to keep your mind on your counting *with extreme gentleness.* This is very important.

- Be patient with yourself.

- Calmly notice anything that comes into your mind.

- When you notice some thought has entered your mind, turn slowly away from it and return to your breathing or counting.

- *Noticing whatever enters your awareness is meditation.*

- *Coming back again and again to your counting is perfect meditation.*

Keep it going:

- Keep at it.

- Use a timer. Sit and meditate at least 1 minute on Day 1, 2 minutes on Day 2, and 3 minutes on Day 3, etc.

- Repeat the above at the same time of day every day.

- Remember: *Be gentle, be patient, and take your time.*

- Increase the minutes at your own pace until you can sit for 20 minutes a day.

- Stick to your routine.

- If you fall off your routine, just start again.

- Remember: You can't fail if you don't quit.

Some helpful tips. Meditation is not a competition or an endurance exercise. Experiment with different chairs and sitting postures so you are upright but comfortable. Gentleness and persistence are the keys.

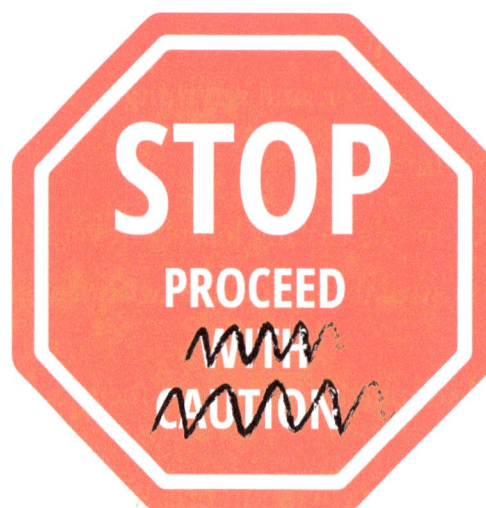

Consciously

The most common problem is trouble paying attention and getting distracted easily. With practice, your attention will improve.

Many beginners make the error of *thinking* about meditation. Meditation is not thinking. It is returning to the breathing or counting whenever you notice you are thinking.

Attentiveness is calming. Distraction is stressful. So stick with it. Being able to calm yourself by returning to your breathing or counting will become easier and easier. And it will become more and more difficult for everyday occurrences and even bigger events to throw you off balance.

Don't take my word for it. Try meditating in this way and decide for yourself. Add it to your recovery routine. But *really* try it. For a few months or, better, for a few years. Then decide. Ultimate Recovery takes time. Remember that it's a journey not a fix. I think you will find it is worth it.

CHAPTER 17

CULTIVATING BIG MIND: THE PRACTICE OF PRESENCE

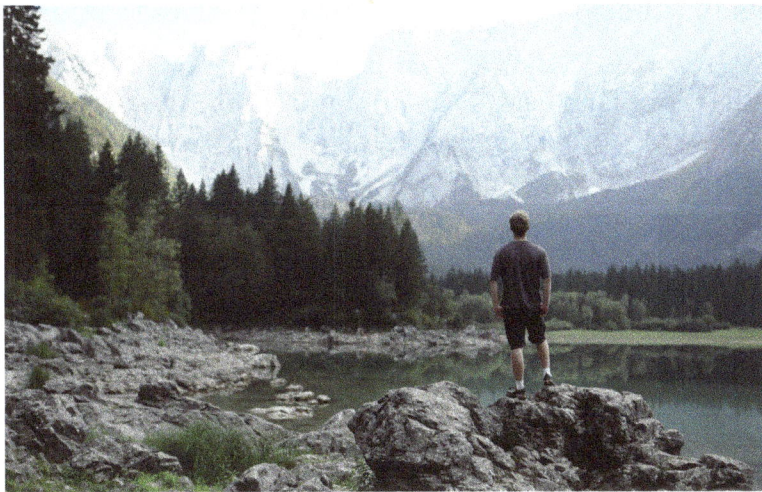

This chapter is a continuation of the ideas developed in the last chapter on the Practice of Serenity. The Practice of Presence is about taking meditation off your seat and out into the world. Let's review.

Our brains are automatic association machines. They churn out thoughts whether we like it or not. The activity in our heads doesn't stop even when we sleep. The constant flow of thoughts, judgments, impressions, insights, and impulses can create needless stress. We relate to this mostly automatic mental activity as something we are doing. But we are no more doing this type of thinking than we are doing the heart beating in our chest or the breathing in our lungs. The amount of intentional, purposeful thinking we do is a mere fraction of the automatic kind.

In this chapter we'll explore how to cultivate an experience of living that is more intentional, realistic, and calm, a state of mind we'll refer to as Big Mind.

Big Mind. By quieting down the automatic activity of our brains, intentionally being still, and calmly observing what is going on around us and in us, we become more aware. Our world opens up. There's more to see, and it's more in perspective. This is what is called Big Mind. Until we practice presence, we tend to have a reactive mind filled with distraction that never stops, which doesn't give us the opportunity to see what's really going on.

Cultivating Big Mind is the solution. Meditation, what I refer to as the Practice of Serenity, is the foundation for Big Mind. In this chapter we'll take it further.

The problem of addiction to our thoughts. As we covered in previous chapters, our mind is a virtual reality machine. It fills our heads with all kinds of mostly random imaginings, both grand and grave, both ecstatic and catastrophic. We may not realize that we may have come to prefer the drama in our head over our actual, average, normal, ordinary life. The "reality" concocted by our mind can seem so much more important.

The dramatic virtual reality concocted by our mind serves to take us away from the normal, average, ordinary, "boring" realities of Life. But is present-mindedness actually boring? This is something we'll explore in this chapter.

There is a payoff for remaining in our head. Permitting our mind to run on automatic may also distract us from the grimmer realities of our life, like our vulnerability and death. This may seem like a good thing. But there is a cost for allowing ourselves to be shielded from these realities. We'll explore this too.

Presence. The words "consciousness," "awareness," and "presence" are basically synonyms. To be conscious is to be aware. To be aware is to be present.

Being fully present is like looking at a picture in an art gallery. When you appreciate a painting, you look at the whole painting more than at any single feature. But we don't typically experience our life as a whole as we do a picture. We instead focus on individual elements. We focus first on this then on that, reacting to each person, each utterance, each event, each situation one at a time. This is like focusing on a single object in a painting one at a time but never taking in the picture as a whole. So the whole of our life is essentially lost on us. What a pity.

Three states of mind. There are three states of mind. The first two states we're familiar with. The scattered, unfocused monkey mind discussed earlier in this book we'll call the absent-minded state. When we're in this state, we are lost in our head. We may be aware of our thoughts but very little of what's actually going on around us.

A second state of mind is the working, focused task-minded state. We typically regard this ability to focus our attention on something as the ultimate state of mind. Focusing our attention provides us with the ability to deal with people and tasks, to relate to others, and to get things done. So this task-minded state is important, but it's not all there is.

The absent-minded and task-minded states have something in common. They both break up reality into pieces as we attend to one thought, one emotion, one sensation, one experience, one conversation, one activity at a time. This distorts the way things actually are. Real life occurs all at once and never stops. When our perception is limited to one thing at a time, we miss a lot.

The third state of mind, the focus of this chapter, may be less familiar. We'll call it present-minded. It involves a high level of consciousness, a high level of awareness. It is a state of mind in which we perceive Life as a whole, as it is—the big picture if you will.

Three States of Mind

	Autopilot, Unfocused, Absent-Minded	Intentional, Focused, Task-Minded	Still, Aware, Present-Minded
General Description	Monkey mind, automatic, undirected, default mode of the brain	Mind at work, brain activity directed at a task	Big Mind, nonreactivity that opens our mind, allowing us to see the big picture
Scope of Awareness	Unpredictable awareness, random thoughts and emotions	Focused awareness narrowed to promote attention to task, topic, person, or situation at hand	Broad, inclusive awareness of whatever is present—thoughts, emotions, body states, surroundings; no single focus; no foreground, no background
What It's Like	Pointless web surfing; a procession of images, ideas, and emotions	Sitting in a well-lit room equipped for a particular type of work	Sitting high, overlooking the countryside, calmly aware of the hustle, the bustle, *and the peace*
Goal of Practice	To reduce this	To sharpen this	To be capable of this

What is present-mindedness good for? Our absent-minded state is automatic and often pointless and stressful. Our task-minded state is vital for performing tasks. Is there a point to present-mindedness? What's it good for? There are several answers to this question: Present-mindedness fosters awareness and promotes the capacity for choice. It is good for our mental and physical health. But perhaps most important, it helps us become more acquainted with Life as it is.

A present-minded state is associated with a more reliable state of calm. The science of mindfulness on which this practice is based makes that evident. As a result, we may enjoy lower blood pressure and better emotional regulation. The latter point is worth expanding upon.

When we get triggered, it's because something or someone seems bigger and more important than everything else. This is because we're focusing on it as if it's the only thing there is in that moment. Present-mindedness allows us to be more aware *of the context of the situations we face.* It allows us to see things in their proper perspective—as one thing among many others, *never as the only thing, never as the biggest thing.*

This allows us to remain calm in situations that used to trigger us. When we see things and people in the context of other events that are also occurring, we are more apt to take things in stride. When we see things against the backdrop of the vastness of our life, there are no, or very few, big things. It brings to mind the saying, "Don't sweat the small stuff—and it's *all* small stuff."

Present-mindedness is not about either sadness or happiness. It's just about being aware there is always more, much more, in every moment than what is making you sad or happy. It's about being aware that your life in every moment is truly vast.

Yet another advantage of present-mindedness is that it facilitates choice. Being present, being aware permits us the ability to see our circumstances more clearly. We are more likely to see possible alternatives and therefore be able to choose among them.

Being present-minded allows us to look before we leap. Without the mind of presence, we may be reactive and reenacting old patterns again and again more or less automatically. Present-mindedness can be a preventive against acting impulsively or out of fear or excitement.

The final advantage may be the biggest of all. Present-mindedness is an antidote for the endless anxiety-ridden seeking many of us engage in. Think of the last time you lost your keys and were looking everywhere to find them. Were you mentally present or were you trying to recall where you might have left them even while your eyes were darting about furiously and/or thinking about how you were going to be late or some other dire consequence?

We spend a lot of our time seeking. What are *you* looking for? A friend? A job? Success? A good place to eat? A better place to live? An escape from boredom? Your keys? Recovery? Happiness? How much of your day would you say you spend looking for, thinking about, wishing for, missing, craving, recalling, or assessing something or someone? When you're engaged in seeking of anything, are you mostly present or mostly lost in your head? Do these kinds of behaviors take up a small or large amount of your day? Be honest.

The point is that if we spend most of our time seeking, we fail to notice the basic goodness of our life as it is in this very moment.

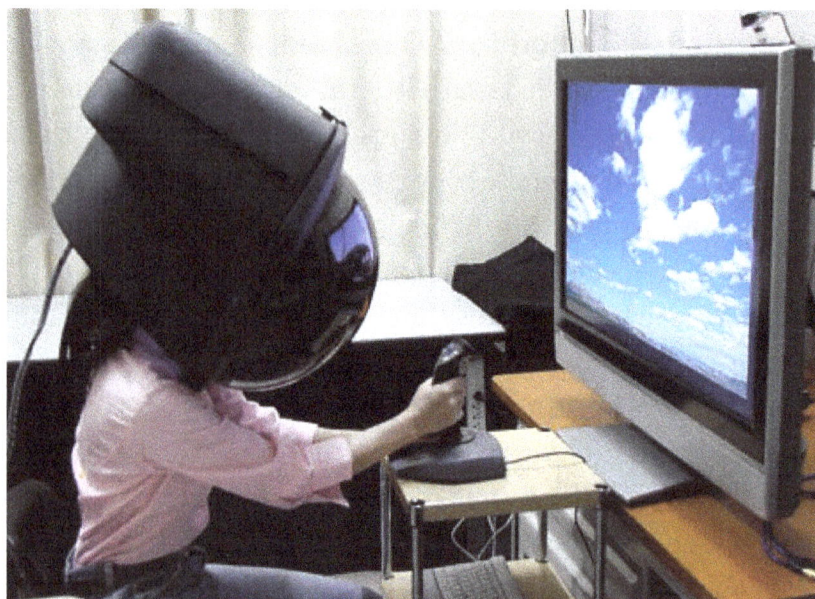

Is there a downside to being present-minded? Being absent-minded may be preferable if you've decided that ordinary life is boring or too grim to bear. Everyone's situation is different, and I don't judge you for how you live your life, but let me briefly suggest a few ideas for your consideration.

If your life feels too boring, I would say, "Wake up!" There is nothing boring about Life if you're really taking it in clearly. "Boring" is a term used when our reality has become clouded and narrowed by attitudes, expectations, and repetitive actions. Once we submit to our virtual reality generator, actual life doesn't stand a chance *unless you can find a way to break through the interference.* As I've said many times, when and if you do break through, you will be amazed at how basically good your normal, average, ordinary life is.

How about the need to escape from grim realities? If you're talking about ultimate realities like old age, sickness, and death, it's no surprise that you would want to avoid facing them. But let's briefly acknowledge the cost of doing so. It is death, the ultimate reality, that instructs us that Life is precious, that each year, month, day, hour, and moment counts. Don't you owe it to yourself to come to know Life fully before you pass on? Only you can answer that question.

We live in a death-denying culture that seeks to prevent us from acknowledging the reality of death—until it's too late. I can tell you only that learning to live with a healthy regard for my own vulnerability and mortality has added more to my life than anything, anything else I have learned.

Death is the ultimate teacher urging us to wake up. I can't say I have no fear of death, but I can say that I no longer live *in fear* of death. I have come to live with a *healthy* regard for my mortality. And I have come to appreciate that I'm not alone. My mortality connects me with *every living being*.

A cautionary tale about living absent-mindedly—driving to work. I was running late for work this morning. I had a forty-minute car ride but only thirty minutes before my first meeting of the day. And what made it worse was that I was the one running the meeting.

It's a simple fact that I was going to be late. I couldn't change the laws of physics. But that didn't stop me from being upset for the whole forty minutes while trying to make up time by employing some questionable driving tactics and, I'm sure, angering and possibly endangering some of my fellow motorists in the process.

Being present-minded requires that we are capable of being aware of what exists at the tip of our senses, taking full notice of what is there rather than trying to bypass it, as I was this day.

But I wasn't able to see my strongly developed mental habits in action, so I couldn't free myself from them. As a result, every second of the drive to work that day was excruciating. It would have been OK for me to do my best to make up time, as long as I didn't put myself or anyone else at risk (I really don't think I did), but in the back of my head was that thought—"If I just push ... hard ... enough, I just ... might ... make it on TIME!!!" In the back of my head was this ridiculous notion that maybe I *could* alter the very physics of time and space.

Had I not gotten so irritated, so caught up in my monkey mind so quickly, I might have relaxed a bit and simply remained present with the simple fact that I would be late. I might still have tried to reduce the degree of my lateness, but I might have done so with a little more composure, grace, and safety awareness. I might not have lost forty or so minutes out of my life to misery, which I created for myself, not just by being late in the first place *but also by how I reacted to it.*

Not only did I ruin my drive to work, raise my heart rate and blood pressure, irritate my fellow motorists, and cause myself to feel generally miserable for almost an hour in the very beginning of my day, but my foul mood and impatience might have caused an accident or spilled over into my meeting, creating a whole new raft of problems.

I am certain that I failed to return a few "good mornings" with any degree of warmth or civility. I may not have heard someone speaking to me at all at first, so lost was I in my mental jungle with my monkeys.

Question: When are you fully awake and entirely unconscious?

Answer: When you're lost in THOUGHT!

The subtle, mysterious Practice of Presence—thinking less, seeing more. Your life and my life are not concepts. Our life is not ideas. Our life doesn't occur in our heads. Reality is only ever what is being played out here, now, in a succession of heres and nows. The playing field is right in front of us, and we're not merely spectators. We are the players!

Would a football player confuse the sports commentary about the game with the actual playing of the game? Of course not. So we have to try to stop confusing the commentary in our heads with what is going on in our actual life, right here, right now.

It's only when we stop the mental chatter that we can fully experience what is happening on the playing field of our life. Here, now. This is the beginning of our Practice of Presence. And it is both subtle and mysterious.

It is subtle because presence requires you to do less and be *more aware*, to think less and *see more*, not just with your eyes but also with your mind. This mental vision is a subtle power of the mind that we rarely take advantage of. It's mysterious because in time, we come to realize just how vast our life is, how limitless it is, how many wonderful moments there are to experience in a normal, average, ordinary moment, hour, day, week, month, and life.

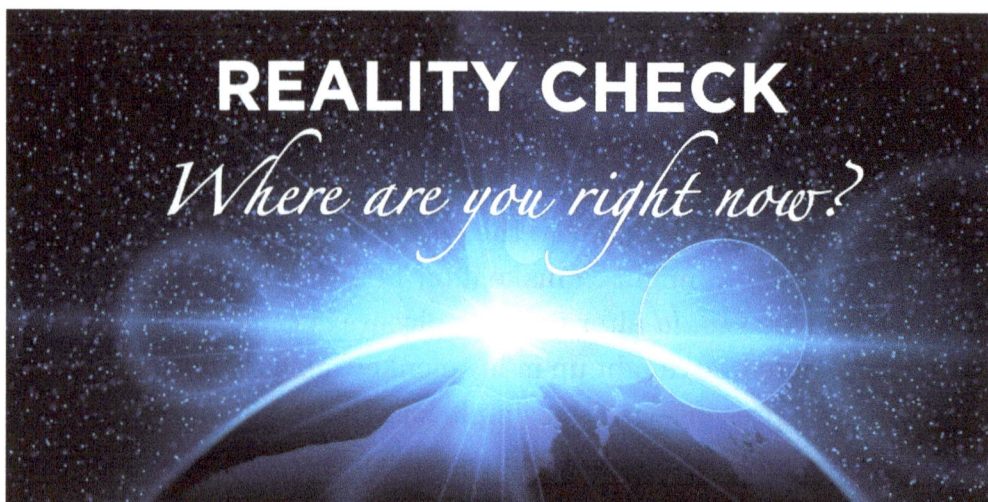

REALITY CHECK
Where are you right now?

Exercise: Grounding in the Present. Take the next 24 hours and see if you can catch yourself going off mentally and creating problems. See if you can catch yourself obsessing over something that is making you angry, sad, regretful, anxious, jealous, uncertain, frightened, or outraged—*something that has no place in the current situation.*

Once you have caught your mind in this way, see if you can bring yourself back to where you are and what you are doing, back to your body, simply noticing what you see, hear, and feel with your hands and feet and on your skin. See if you can stay with the present moment for a few seconds or even a minute at a time. You may discover that you have a very hard time staying with anything for this long. *You may begin to realize how rarely you are present in your life.*

See if you can catch yourself being lost in your head. Then bring yourself back, the best you can, to the present moment, to your body, as I described above. Decide if it felt different to be present compared with being off somewhere in your mind. Write a few lines describing the difference.

_____

_____

_____

Lean in. The Practice of Realism we covered earlier in this book is about clearing your head of unrealistic attitudes and expectations. It is about accepting the *idea of reality*. The Practice of Presence is learning to *live in reality*. If you can take on this subtle and mysterious Practice of Presence and train yourself to lean in and connect with what you are doing and who you are doing it with; more and more often, you will find that you feel more grounded and that you are often quite content.

Once again, there's nothing wrong with thinking. We need to do it to perform important activities that support our lives. But we don't need to spend all of our time in our head. The Practice of Presence is about achieving balance and not confusing our thoughts—our commentary on our life, our analysis, our worries, our hopes—with the real thing. Does it make sense that the more you can practice being present—and not lost in thoughts about the past, present, or future—the more you may come to simply appreciate your life as it is?

This moment is your life.
If you miss it, you miss everything.

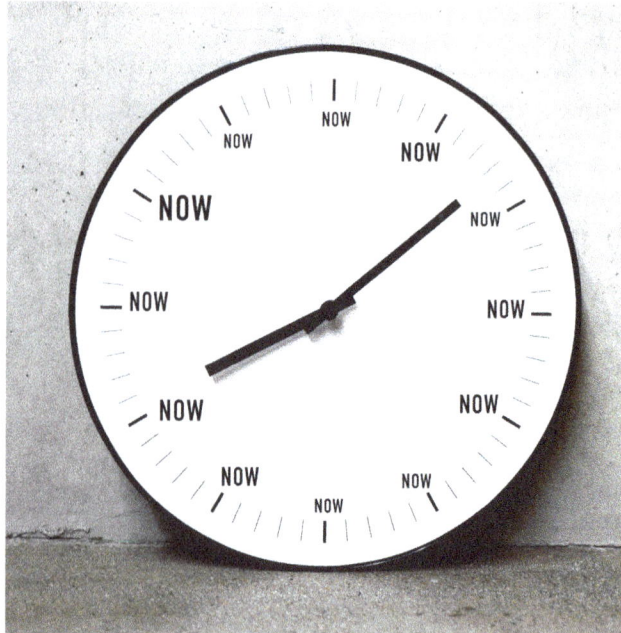

How often can you afford to miss everything?

Stillness in motion. Without stillness of mind, and the clarity that comes with it, we react incessantly, automatically, impulsively—first to this and then to that, pulling this idea, that emotion, this sight or sound, this experience, this concern, etc., up close to us. Whenever we do this, we distort the importance of the particulars of our life by blocking out the bigger picture. We become confined in a small space that is a miniscule part of our here and now—whenever and wherever we may be.

A thinking view of Life is a nearsighted one. We notice trees but never forests. We hear notes but never music. We see a brushstroke or two, a fragment or two of an image, but we never see the full picture.

The stillness and vision we acquire in the seated meditation of the Practice of Serenity are what we can learn to take with us into our daily life. This taking stillness along with us, wherever we go, into each moment of our life, is the Practice of Presence, known also as mindfulness.

Mindfulness is stillness in motion. Consider the following:

- Can you compose a text on your phone with such focus that you lose track of everything else?

- Can you, after learning to experience stillness, compose the same text with a calm, quiet mind, without losing track of everything else, maintaining a larger awareness even while you focus on your texting?

- The answer to both questions is yes.

- *Which is more real?*

- Can you address your child's behavior with such focus you lose track of everything else?

- Can you, after learning to experience stillness, address the same situation with a calm, attentive mind, with awareness that this situation is only one thing happening among many others even while you interact with your child?

- The answer to both is again, yes, of course.

- *Which is more real?*

- Can you do a job with such intense focus that you lose track of everything else?

- Can you bring some stillness to the job and practice not losing track of the rest of your life and maintaining perspective even while you perform efficiently and well?

- Yes again to both.

- *Again, which is more real?*

- Can you do your best to plan for the future with such focus and fear that you lose track of everything else?

- Can you, with practice, do your best to plan for your future with greater stillness, without losing track of everything else, maintaining a larger awareness, keeping the planning in perspective, and thereby approaching this task more calmly?

- Yes!

- *And again, which is more real?*

Without the Practice of Presence, we miss out on our lives as they actually are. By allowing our monkey mind to be in control or by engaging our task mind with excessive busyness, we are focusing only on this or that. We are removed from the flow and wholeness of our life. This may be necessary if we are engaged in an important task like a have-to or a love-to. But if we're always distracted or always busy, it's important to realize we lose moments that become minutes, that become hours, that become days, and so on. If we do this enough, we lose out on our lives.

If we permit it, our monkey mind alone can rob us of our precious life and replace it with distorted ideas, distorted emotions, and needless worry, fear, and hopelessness, all of which stem from feeling trapped by the tiny circumstances we imagine rather than experiencing the spaciousness, freedom, and basic goodness that are our birthright.

Another cautionary tale about living absentmindedly—a story about Bob. The ideas we form about things that happen and the people in our life result in attitudes we have about those things and people. We believe our ideas and our attitudes. We feel they are justified, and perhaps they are. But that's never the whole story.

Our beliefs and attitudes are major obstacles to becoming present-minded. We can't avoid developing beliefs and attitudes. We acquire them—*positive and negative ones*—about just about everything. Earlier we referred to this as our programming. Our belief and attitude programming is hard to change. But to experience our life as it actually is, we have to be capable of seeing beyond our programming, of breaking through this interference so we can see people, places, and things in our life as they actually are rather than how we *think* they are, rather than how we think they *should* be, rather than how we *expect* them to be.

We've talked about the incessant activity in our head that occurs throughout every day. When we're dealing with other people, especially those we have some history with, the monkeys can go into overdrive! Here's an example of someone who is trapped, and possibly trapping others, in their attitudes. Let's see if you can relate.

Bob walks by. Mary doesn't like Bob based on some things he has done in the past. Mary feels justified in feeling the way she does. In other words, she feels justified in having the *attitude* she has toward him. And perhaps she is. But Bob is nice today. In fact, Bob has been nice for a while. Bob has had some experiences recently that have helped him realize he hasn't been a nice person in the past, and now he wants to change. He *is* changing. Bob is happier, and other people are happier around him. People who know Bob are taking notice. But not Mary.

Because of her past experiences, her conditioning, her programming, she doesn't notice, or she decides that this new behavior isn't *real*, that he's being a phony and she can't trust him. This is what she has come to believe. Perhaps it's wise to be cautious with Bob based on her past experience. But won't it be a shame if Bob really has changed, or is trying to, and it turns out that Mary is the one making it difficult for him to change his future because of attitudes and beliefs she has formed? In a way, both Mary and Bob are trapped by them.

Have you experienced anything like this? Have you made up stories about someone that prevent you from seeing the whole person? Do you think others have done this to you?

Isn't the fact that you are reading this book an indication that *you* are making a change in your life? Do you want people you know and care about to be open to these changes and support you? I expect you do. But you may find some of these people have old ideas about you—old attitudes, old beliefs—that make it hard for them to see and honor the changes you are making. Because of this, you feel they don't support you. They are trapped by their programming, and if you're not careful, you can be trapped by it as well.

Attitudes and beliefs close our mind from seeing anything new. Attitudes and beliefs keep us from letting go of the past and being present to what is actually occurring. They keep us from being realistic, from being able to see what is real, what is here and now. Being realistic means being able to see beyond your programming and realize that what was true in the past may no longer be true.

It's hard to see beyond our programming but not impossible. The first step is to realize you have attitudes and beliefs, and the second is to try to step back from them, quiet your mind, and see what is actually going on here and now. This is what it means to be present. It means quieting our mind a bit throughout every day, so we can see more clearly what is going on in the situation we are in, free of what we expect to see, and thereby let go of the past and possibly establish new, healthier relationships and healthier patterns of living our life.

Presence is how we see the constant newness each moment brings. When someone says, "Nothing ever changes," that's a tip-off that they're trapped in their programming and cut off from what's really going on. In fact, many of us believe that little ever changes. In truth, everything does, constantly. Moment to moment we are presented with endless opportunities to choose new approaches to our life.

But you can't become present by talking or reading about it. Whatever you can say about it, it won't help you experience it. Just like talking about food will never give you the sensation of taste, talking about presence isn't going to help you be present.

A lesson from the martial arts. Did you ever wonder how a martial artist reacts so quickly to the rapid movements of their opponent that come from every direction? Is it because they are rapidly scanning their opponent's body and trying to catch the movement of an arm or a leg coming in their direction?

The answer is no, of course not. They do not look at arms and legs and hope their eyes happen to be in the right place at the right time. That would spell disaster. Martial artists are trained to fix their gaze on a single spot of their opponent's body to open up their peripheral vision. *It is the stillness of their gaze that allows their field of vision to open.*

Just as the martial artist keeps his or her eyes calmly fixed on one spot of their opponent's body, thus opening their field of vision so they see every move the opponent makes, we can train our mind to be fixed on a single "spot," for example, on our breathing, and so become more calm and still. *In this way we can open our field of awareness* and see more of what is actually going on in any particular moment so we can respond appropriately to it.

Through such training we can transform a life that seems boring and trivial, and that makes some individual things seem huge and overwhelming, into a here and now that is vast and rich, where everything changes, and where everything is in its proper perspective. We can become more and more able to calmly see what is present, accurately and completely. Like the martial artist, because we see all, we become more and more able to respond to our circumstances whatever they may be.

During seated meditation we practice sustaining a mental image of our breath, keeping our mental gaze fixed there, calmly, so we are able to see the panorama of the present that includes many things—a thought, a twinge in our belly, an emotion, a recollection, a sound, a worry, a plan—all of it, allowing all of it in, realizing it is all ours, it is all Life, it is all *our* life. Everything is important in its own way, but no one thing is more important than any other, *and no one thing is remotely as big as this moment.*

Through seated meditation our reality opens up and over time becomes vast. We experience a sense of freedom, an absence of restraint. The fear, anxiety, and claustrophobia dissipate. We breathe more easily. We become capable of responding with ease, genuineness, and warmth.

Once again, the Practice of Presence is taking meditation off the seat and into our lives. This is the beginning of wisdom. And it is yours if you want it. You can't fail if you don't quit practicing.

Try it. The Practice of Presence may be the most powerful and most challenging of the practices in this book. Start by practicing the simple instructions that follow. We'll approach this practice gradually in small, bite-size steps.

The Practice of Presence Part 1: Warm Up. Do this before engaging with other people or beginning any task.

Pause: Stop and take a breath.

Presence: Take it all in. Be aware of what is happening in the moment; notice thoughts, feel emotions, experience body sensations, and take in your surroundings. *Stay present with and accepting of whatever arises* just as it is, moment by moment without any big reactions.

Proceed slowly: And be mindful of what you do and say. Respond with care to whatever or whomever needs your attention.

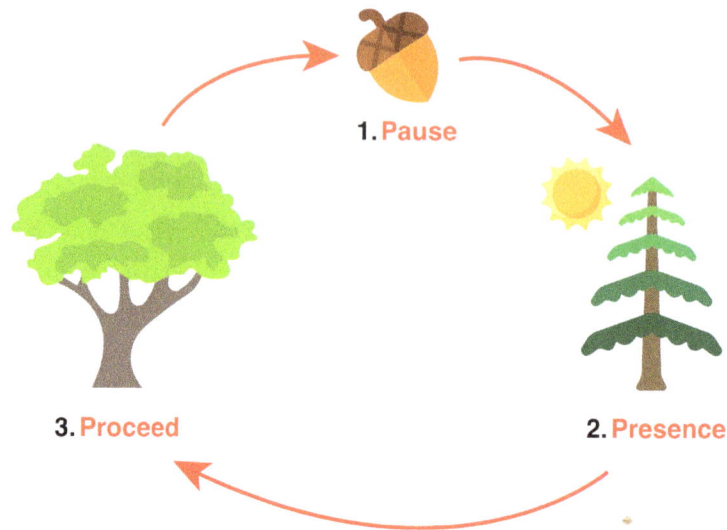

1. Pause

2. Presence

3. Proceed

Stick with this pause-presence-proceed formula for the next 24 hours, then write about what you experience in a paragraph or two. Do this thoughtfully before reading on. Doing this is your commitment to being happier and healthier.

The Practice of Presence Part 2: Daily Guided Meditation. This is a guided meditation. Record it or have someone record it for you so you can listen to it and take it in deeply.

Sit quietly with your feet flat on the floor (as you can).
Put everything out of your hands. Sit as straight and tall as you can,
not leaning left or right, forward or back;
align your left ear over your left shoulder,
your right ear over your right shoulder,
your nose over your belly button,
your hands loose in your lap.
Close your eyes.

Focus on your breathing.
See with your mind the movement of your breathing.
See the in breath, beginning to end.
See the out breath, beginning to end.
See with your mind every second, every movement
of the in and out breaths very carefully.

(Pause)

Keep your mind's eye open, gazing calmly, allowing any thoughts to come and go
but never taking your "eye" off the breath.
In and out. In and out.

(Pause)

Now, while you continue to do this, also see yourself sitting, breathing, with your mind.

(Pause)

Now, while you continue to see your breathing, and see yourself breathing,
also see with your mind the room you are in.

(Pause)

Now, while you continue to see your breathing, and you continue to see
yourself breathing, and seeing yourself sitting in the room you are in,
see with your mind the building you are in too.

(Pause)

Really try to see this.

(Pause)

Now, while you continue to see your breathing with your mind,
move once around the room.
If the room is small, move out of it and then
come back and take your place again.

Continue to see yourself breathing, yourself sitting, and
the environment of the room, and include any physical sensations,
thoughts, and feelings, all as a single mental image.

(Pause)

Sit for at least 1 more minute.

Do this daily guided meditation for up to a week before moving on to Part 3.

The Practice of Presence Part 3: Presence During Quiet Activities. Pick some common quiet activity, such as getting showered and dressed, eating, exercising, doing laundry, cooking, painting, or playing cards. While you are participating in the activity, bring yourself back again and again to your breathing, following your in breaths and out breaths. As best you can, follow your breathing *while* you are doing the activity. It will probably be very difficult at first, and you will have to be patient. Stick with it.

Do this exercise at least once a day and write about it afterward on 4 consecutive days. Answer these questions:

1. Were you able to come all the way back to your breath during the activity? Or did you stay halfway between a focus on your breath and some thought, emotion, or the activity itself? Describe this experience.

2. Did you truly focus on your breath, *following* the inhale and *following* the exhale? Or were you instead thinking about whether it was helping or not or about something else? Describe this experience.

3. If you were successful at following a few breaths, did you feel more in the moment? Write what it was like for you.

4. If you felt more in the moment, did you notice more during the activity? If so, how did that feel?

5. Do you think this exercise is of value? Why or why not?

Practice of Presence Part 4: All Day, Every Day. Go about your business. Do what you would normally do. But try to reserve some attention to keep track of your breathing and your body and to visualize yourself as you do whatever it is you are doing. Practice moving through your day this way.

You will get the best results by practicing seated meditation (Practice of Serenity) for about 20 minutes each day. By combining the practices of Serenity and Presence you will stretch your mind and begin to create a mental mirror within which to see yourself and your present. You will be developing Big Mind.

Be patient. With daily practice you will get better at it. Some days will be better than others. If you are frustrated at times, be present with that too. Allow in whatever it is that is present for you. It's all good, because it's all your life.

Keep practicing and you will get better at keeping things, all things, in perspective by not getting lost in your head. *Nothing—no one, no problem, no thought, no feeling, no situation, no fortune, and no calamity—is bigger than your life.* And everything is temporary. Including you and me.

Remember that exercising Big Mind and being present with the big picture of what is going on here and now doesn't mean pushing anything away. Allow everything in, even the yucky stuff—pain, regret, shame even. But don't focus on any of it.

Part of learning how to deal with painful emotions is to start by just seeing them and allowing them in. *When we can do that, we may discover that they too pass.* Everything passes eventually. Everything. If we let it.

As you become better and better at maintaining perspective, you will become calmer, more confident, less fearful, better able to handle what comes, better able to let go, to be totally present with each new moment, and just be. In this state you will manage your daily activities and relationships with greater peace and effectiveness.

Comparison of the Practices of Serenity and Presence

This table will help you see the similarities and differences between the companion practices of the Practice of Serenity (meditation) and the Practice of Presence (mindfulness).

	Practice of Serenity	Practice of Presence
Known as	Meditation	Mindfulness
Practiced	While sitting down, without distractions	During your regular activities
Purpose	To open the seeing mind by stilling the thinking mind	
Technique	Each time you become aware that you're thinking, come back to the breath.	

	Practice of Serenity	Practice of Presence
Why It Works		Once you become *aware* of thought, you're no longer *lost* in thought. Like the martial artist opening their *field of vision* by focusing on a single spot, focusing on the breath has this effect on our *field of awareness*. You're able to *see* your thought as one *among many things*.
Result		The intended result of practice is an expanded field of awareness that isn't dominated by thinking. You think less but see more, become more aware/present/conscious. You see things *more realistically*, each thing as one among many things happening, the big picture, Big Mind. You no longer perceive your life one thing at a time, so *no one thing dominates your attention or influences your behavior*.
Tips		This can be exhausting work. Do it for short periods and build up. At first it may interfere with your activities. It will definitely interfere with your thinking. But you're probably thinking too much! Over time it will become more natural to see more, think less.

Note: Remember that practice doesn't make perfect. There is no such thing as being perfectly present. Practice is perfect. If you're practicing, you'll improve.

Presence versus happiness. If you think of happiness as exciting, then happiness can't be normal. In order for something to be exciting, it has to be beyond the normal, average, and ordinary in some way. So an excited happiness isn't normal. It's not sustainable either, not without resorting to something unhealthy.

Many people have this notion of excited happiness and have it as their goal in their life to be as constantly "up" as they can be. Unless they are up, they feel like there is something wrong with them or wrong with their lives. Looking to be always up is what gets people hooked on empty experiences like video games, shopping, gambling, sex, alcohol, and drugs, to give just a few examples.

Healthy happiness. Healthy happiness is about *engaging* and *connecting with* what is here and now, not resenting or resisting, not attaching to or pursuing, just being fully present with things as they are. Healthy happiness is about savoring the basic goodness that is often apparent to us when we do this. Being aware of everything—the simple act of brushing our teeth, the comfortable feel of a jacket, easy movement down a hallway, the coolness of a drink of water, a smile, the sound of night. The possibilities for experiencing this kind of basic goodness are endless for the person capable of being present.

Learning to be present even *with uncomfortable feelings* leads us to realize just how impermanent and undramatic most unpleasant feelings and conditions really are—as long as we allow ourselves to fully experience them, *without any big reaction and without holding on to them*. When we are grounded in the present, it is impossible to hold on to anything. Everything is just passing through.

No big thing. Most of what we physically experience in the present is basically good. It's usually remembered or imagined experiences that lead to discontent. The present is subtly happy not excitingly so. Our mental and emotional reactions may create discontent when we build up experiences into something they are not because we are trying to satisfy some idea we have.

Again, what happens to our problems when we drop our thoughts about them? All that remains is what we are taking in and feeling that moment. And what we are taking in and feeling in any moment changes constantly. It all just passes through. For a person living in the present, *everything* is passing through. The landscape is always changing. Nothing ever stays the same.

We may have the habit of building up feelings, especially those we like, to be bigger and more than they are. By grasping on to something about our circumstances and letting our thinking dramatize that, our circumstances and feelings come to feel quite real, quite solid and significant. When we drop our thoughts and just allow our feelings and circumstances to speak for themselves and to pass through, we discover that nothing is so dramatic, that everything is impermanent and not at all solid.

Quiet, ordinary, flowing goodness. Feelings we don't like would tend to go away if we didn't make such a big deal of them and fight with them or try so hard to escape them. Life always moves on. We need to learn to not get stuck in our ideas and to move with them. When we make a big deal out of things that happen by making up stories we tell ourselves again and again, we take ourselves out of the flow of Life and deprive ourselves of its simple goodness.

If we can stop or slow down the commentary in our head and return again and again to our breath, we can experience Life as it actually is—its ups and downs but mostly drama-free and ordinary with lots of basically good moments.

Another cautionary tale—driving home. I was leaving work one day. I was feeling good. By the time I got into my car I was daydreaming about how good I was feeling. I realized I was savoring the moment. Nothing wrong with that, of course, but I realized I was leaving the here and now and starting to make a big deal about feeling good *and trying to make it last.*

Reality had moved on. I had not. I was getting bogged down in my mind.

I'm an occasional cigar smoker, and a few minutes later I asked myself if I should stop and buy a cigar for the ride home. But I realized a moment later that once again, I was looking for something to make the moment even better than it was.

I was recalling how good a good cigar tasted and trying to figure out how to reclaim this experience. While I was doing this in my head, reality moved on. I had taken myself out of the here and now to look for a little more, a little extra pleasure—trying to make a bigger deal out of the basic goodness of the moment that was now passed.

Why did I do this? I teach this stuff. The simple answer: habit. Like most of us, I have a history of confusing excited happiness with healthy quiet happiness, and it still gets the better of me at times. But less than it once did.

And to my credit, I realized what I was doing. I succeeded in letting go of the cigar idea and climbed out of my head. During the next twenty minutes or so of my car ride, I put effort into trying to be present with what I was seeing as I drove down the road without thinking too much. I felt calm, good, just taking it all in, not getting hung up on anything in particular, not lingering on any sight, not thinking, just observing. No big thing. Just basic, ordinary happiness. Subtle. Mysteriously wonderful. It was a good twenty minutes.

It came to me that I should take a picture of the clouds. They were particularly beautiful. Nothing wrong with this either, of course, but there it was again. I was going back into my head. Why did I want to take a picture? To make the experience last. And *once again*, to the credit of my years of practice, I realized I had left the here and now and was thinking—thinking about rather than living my life. Thinking about how to make the moment last. Life had moved on. I got out of my head and moved on with it. I never fail at being present because I never quit working at it.

A moment cannot last no matter what we do, except in our mind. We try to stop the flow and create some feeling of permanence by mentally holding on to the good times and mentally trying to move ourselves past the bad ones. But by doing this, we (1) expend an awful lot of effort, (2) take ourselves out of the reality of here and now, (3) may never come to appreciate the basic quiet goodness of our life, and (4) assure our own misery by setting ourselves the impossible task of making what we like last and making what we dislike vanish.

When I arrived home, I noticed I had a text message from a friend with a YouTube attached. It was a video of a magician making a playing card disappear in an amazing way.

It occurred to me that we're all magicians in a way. All of us have the ability to make reality vanish. How? By getting into our heads and joining the monkeys. And all of us have the ability to make thoughts and feelings vanish. How? By being present.

Whatever is bothering you will vanish if you simply allow yourself to be present with what you're feeling instead of trying to get past it. This may seem contradictory, but it's true. Feelings don't last. Only our thoughts about them do. If we can train ourselves to be truly present, we can come to experience that again and again.

Trying to make bad feelings go away gives them a life in our mind that they do not have without our help. In our mind we dramatize and prolong our bad feelings. By thinking about our bad feelings and saying to ourselves things like, "Damn, I feel lousy. Why am I feeling this way? I need to do something to take my mind off this," we give life to a phantom and neglect the life before us.

A final tale—my airport epiphany. An experience I once had at an airport really helped me appreciate the value of the practices in this book.

I had to be to the airport for a 7 a.m. flight. It was Sunday and I was returning to New York from a professional conference in Orlando, Florida. The shuttle service insisted that I needed to leave my hotel by 3:30 a.m. to get to the airport and through all the security checks in time for my flight. I took their word for it and set my alarm for 2:30 a.m. That would give me enough time to shower, dress, and finish packing.

As luck would have it, there was no traffic. I was at the airport by 4 a.m. Security was a breeze, and I was through all the checks by 4:15. I had almost three hours to kill! I was tired, and I was grumpy.

Thankfully, there was a coffee shop open. I got myself a cup and sat down to surf the internet on my iPad. At 5 a.m. a gift shop opened. I sauntered in to peruse the merchandise. Immediately inside the front door was a rack of T-shirts with the logo "Life is Good."

I had an immediate reaction. I was thinking that Life wasn't so good at this ungodly hour. And wondering what I was thinking agreeing to such an early ride to the airport. And how incompetent the shuttle dispatcher was doling out such ridiculous advice. And …

I stopped.

I realized I was heading into a downward spiral and picking up speed. I could feel that my body was tensing up, and I was prepping myself to be miserable. I took a breath. I widened my gaze and looked around. I very consciously felt my hands in my pockets and my feet on the floor. I came back to the present.

A thought flashed through my mind. "I'm not sick. I'm not bleeding. I'm not cold or starving. I'm perfectly safe. And in a minute or two another group of shops is about to open. I need to get some little thing for my wife anyway."

Several years of practice were paying off at this very moment.

Exercise: The Rest of Your Life. Start off in the morning with a minute to 20 minutes of silent meditation. Then sit quietly a moment longer. Before you do anything else, relax your body, relax your mind, and observe your breathing and every sensation you are aware of. Just sit, nothing more, for at least 1 whole minute. Then for the rest of the day, try the following simple exercise.

Try to be present with the common activities and people you spend time with at each hour of the next 24 hours.

- Slow down.

- Be aware of your body.

- Be aware of your breath.

- Focus completely on what you're doing right now.

- Be aware of thoughts that take you away from the present moment.

- Notice the unremarkable—the floor, walls, the feel of your clothing, the ceiling, the ground outside, smells, a blade of grass, etc.

- Pay particularly close attention when you bathe, groom, dress, and eat.

- Be aware of silence. Brief silences occur in some of the noisiest environments.

- Pay even closer attention whenever you come in contact with another person.

- Silently welcome him or her into your presence.

- Take careful notice of their eyes.

- Hold eye contact for a second or two longer than you typically do.

- Be aware of any judgments that arise; judgments lead to thinking and story-making that take you away.

- Take a walk in nature whenever you can.

- Feel Life around you. You are that Life too!

FINAL WORDS AND WHAT TO DO WHEN THINGS COME APART

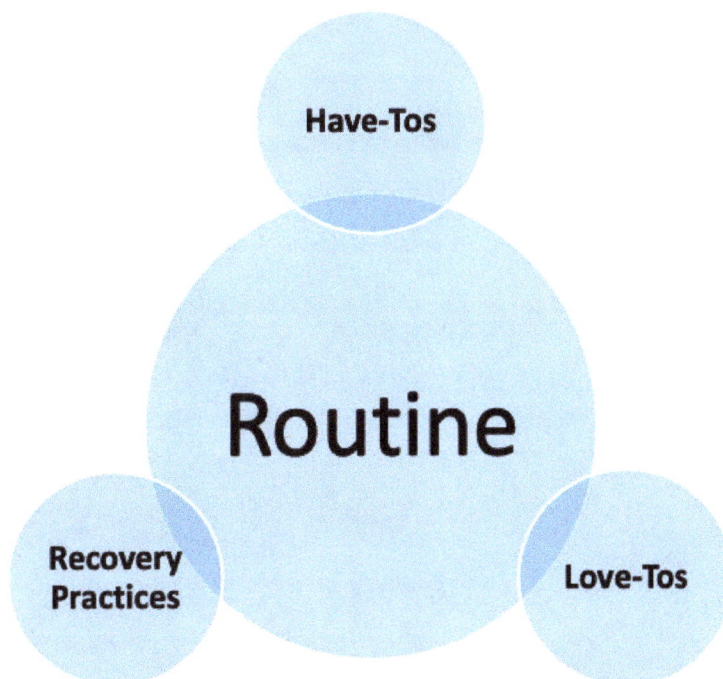

Have-Tos

Routine

Recovery Practices

Love-Tos

Review. Ultimate Recovery begins with understanding that Life is unpredictable, uncontrollable, and ever-changing. Your injury is one example of this, but there are many examples in everyone's life if we stop and think about them. And although it's true that we can't control the circumstances of our life, we *can* control how we live with those circumstances.

How a person lives is what we call lifestyle. Managing our lifestyle according to the principles of Ultimate Recovery is a lifestyle that will lead you to achieving and maintaining your best mental and physical health. Ultimate Recovery will thus provide you with the most solid foundation for achieving other goals that are important to you.

Best mental and physical health is the result of living by a routine organized around three main life activities: things we *have* to do, things we *love* to do, and the *7 Recovery Practices*. Each component of this formula is vital, and each supports and strengthens the others. There is no perfecting any of them; there is only practice. As I have said many times throughout this book, "Practice *is* perfection." You can't fail if you never quit practicing.

How to Recover Again and Again. The Ultimate Recovery lifestyle is also the way to right the boat after being capsized by one of Life's unpredictable waves. It is a remedy or antidote for the various poisons that Life may bring. If a tree falls on my house tonight, the only things I'm going to be thinking about are keeping my dogs from escaping through the shattered wall, keeping the weather out, and calling my insurance company (and hoping I'm covered). Then I'll have to find a reputable contractor who will do the repair job right at the best price in the shortest amount of time. The last thing on my mind will be my routine of have-tos, love-tos, and the 7 Recovery Practices!

Our life is always shifting under our feet, throwing us off balance due to both pleasant and unpleasant events occurring out of the blue, making it challenging to keep our balance and move forward. In such circumstances all we need to do is realize that we're off our routine and that it's not a catastrophe—as long as we get back to it at some point. If we have made it a priority in our life to practice a healthy lifestyle, getting back on track will be easier.

It also helps to remind yourself that making your best mental and physical health a priority is the least selfish thing you can do. It is the foundation of anything else you may want to accomplish in your life, including supporting others. Your best you is the greatest gift you can give those you love.

In my experience, people fail to achieve their goals not because they don't want them badly enough. They fail at achieving goals because they don't remain focused or because when they set them aside due to circumstances beyond their control, they don't remember to pick them back up again. It may help to wear some article of jewelry, like a wrist bracelet, that will remind you of your commitment to best mental and physical health and the practices in this book.

Remember that you are embarking on a change of lifestyle and that such a dramatic change must happen over a lifetime. So pace yourself. Re-read and re-reflect often. Expect obstacles and difficulty along the way. But there is no rush, the practice itself is the objective, not some notion of perfection. The long-term rewards will be substantial if you will just commit to taking your time and to not quitting.

My final gift to you is the Recovery Wheel, below. Make a copy of it and post it somewhere conspicuous in your home. Frame it even. Most of the time when things aren't going well, it is because we have been neglecting one or more of the components. The Recovery Wheel will help you get back on track by making it easier to recall the components of Ultimate Recovery.

Following the Recovery Wheel is My Daily Recovery Wheel Invocation. I encourage you to recite it every day. It is a way of reaffirming your commitment to your Ultimate Recovery lifestyle and maintaining your motivation to keep it up.

You can't fail if you don't quit.
THE RECOVERY WHEEL

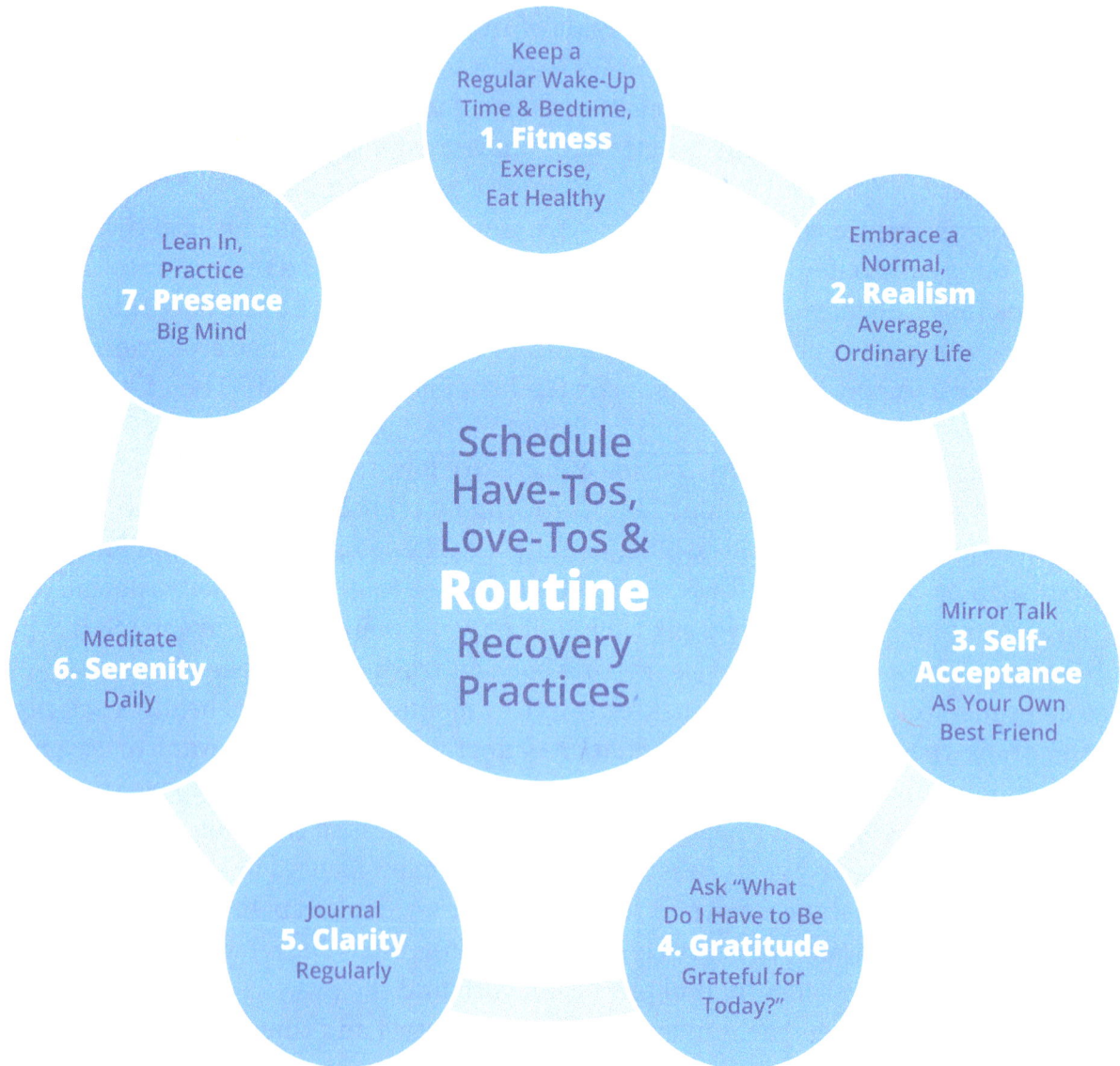

Keep a Regular Wake-Up Time & Bedtime,
1. Fitness
Exercise, Eat Healthy

Embrace a Normal,
2. Realism
Average, Ordinary Life

Lean In, Practice
7. Presence
Big Mind

Schedule Have-Tos, Love-Tos & **Routine** Recovery Practices

Mirror Talk
3. Self-Acceptance
As Your Own Best Friend

Meditate
6. Serenity
Daily

Journal
5. Clarity
Regularly

Ask "What Do I Have to Be
4. Gratitude
Grateful for Today?"

You become what you practice. Everything you need to create an Ultimate Recovery lifestyle is right here. Commit to turning this Recovery Wheel every day.

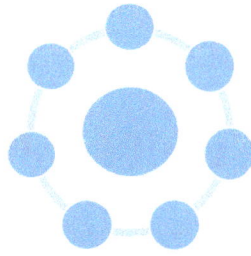

My Daily Recovery Wheel Invocation

Routine

I promise myself to go to sleep at the same time every night so I can wake up at the same time every day. This is the basis of routine. Then I will schedule some have-tos, love-tos, and Recovery Practices—and stick to my schedule.

Fitness

I promise myself to report any regular sleep disturbance to my doctor, to eat and drink in moderation, and to have a scheduled exercise program that I stick to.

Realism

I promise myself to embrace a normal, average, ordinary life and to expect a little boredom, joy, and suffering. My Ultimate Recovery lifestyle will tend to balance these extremes.

Self-Acceptance

I promise myself to check with myself in the mirror each day, to want to know how I feel, and to listen to and regard my feelings with dignity and respect. I will ask myself how I feel, and I will listen to my answer. I will accept my answer and myself as OK, whatever I feel.

Gratitude

Today, I am grateful for … (I will think of something every day).

Clarity

I promise myself to face a blank page of my journal, once a week, and to fill it with what's on my mind. I will wait patiently for something to come and will write it down.

Serenity

I promise myself to spend at least 20 minutes a day in sitting meditation.

Presence

I promise myself to return to my breath throughout the day and allow more of Life in, never limiting myself to what I'm thinking about or doing. My life is bigger. Always bigger.

You deserve your best mental and physical health.
Those you love deserve you at your best.
You will become what you practice.
Practice is perfect.

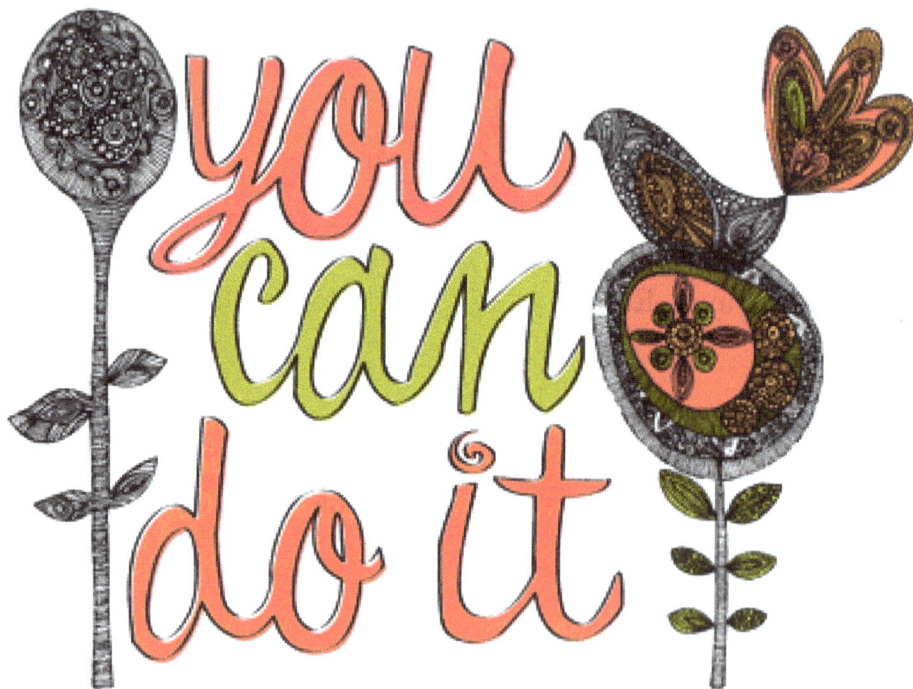

You can't fail
If you don't quit.

AUTHOR BIO

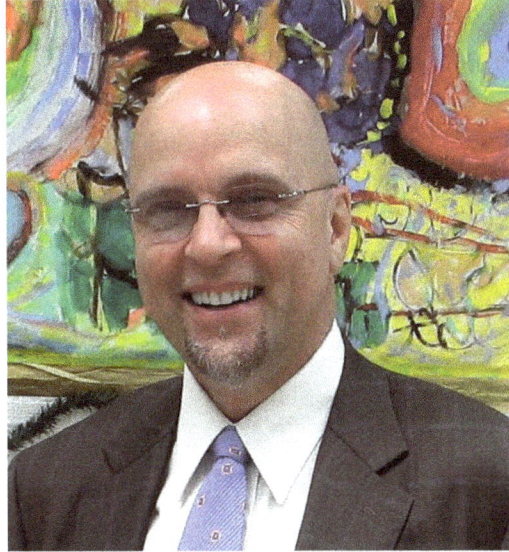

Gerry Brooks began his career in private practice in 1979 as a licensed speech-language pathologist, specializing in cognitive and communicative disorders. He has logged thousands of treatment hours with survivors of brain injury and their families, and served as a consultant to hospitals, rehabilitation centers, and school systems.

In 1998 Gerry joined the planning team for the Northeast Center for Rehabilitation & Brain Injury in Lake Katrine, New York, a year prior to its opening and served as the center's program director until his retirement in 2023. He was responsible in that time for the development and oversight of the center's neurorehabilitation and neurobehavioral programs. Gerry has presented on various brain injury topics at state, national, and international venues.

Gerry has a master's degree in speech-language pathology, and during his career he has held the certificate of clinical competence by the American Speech-Language-Hearing Association, the certified brain injury specialist trainer credential from the Brain Injury Association of America, the technical trainer certification from The Mandt System of therapeutic behavioral support, and a contemplative care certificate from the New York Zen Center for Contemplative Care.

His primary interests are meditation, tennis, motivation, self-awareness, and life-long well-being.

* 9 7 9 8 2 1 8 4 5 4 2 3 4 *